A Diet To Stop Arthritis

....

The Nightshades And Ill Health

Our Goal

To help find the causes of human health problems associated with nutrition. The combined efforts will be needed of the medical and agricultural researchers together with 1000s of willing cooperators.

The Cover: The nightshades that may cause health problems with people, at first subtle and later serious, include *tobacco, tomatoes* of all kinds — cherry, plum, green, yellow, red; *peppers* of all kinds (except black and white), including pimiento, chili, red, green, hot, sweet; the *eggplant* of all sizes, shapes and colors; the *white potato* regardless of skin color; and any of the *processed products* of these crops.

A Diet To Stop Arthritis

The Nightshades and Ill Health

By

NORMAN FRANKLIN CHILDERS, PhD

Blake Professor of Horticulture,
Cook College, Rutgers University, New Jersey
Ass't Director and Sr. Plant Physiologist
U.S. Dept. of Agriculture in Puerto Rico
Associate in Horticulture, Ohio State University
Instructor in Pomology, Cornell University, New York

Please Order Books From

HORTICULTURAL PUBLICATIONS
Somerset Press, Inc., Somerville, N.J. 08876

Phone: 201-722-3000
Send check or money order, $9.95

(Most of book money will be
used to continue research)

By

Norman F. Childers, Publisher

U.S. Library of Congress
Catalogue Card No. 80-83441
ISBN 9-938378-00-7

Printed By
Somerset Press, Inc.
Somerville, New Jersey 08876
Cover and Binding by Horowitz and Son,
Fairfield, New Jersey 07006.

Contents

Thanks

To the thousands of cooperators who helped with the results presented in this book.

Preface, Second Edition

Many people have asked for a paperback of the first edition of this book at less cost. This we have done. The first edition was probably too technical. Most references and technical language have been eliminated in this edition. Chapters have been shortened. If a reader desires an in-depth study, please contact your local library for a first edition or contact the author.

About 5000 copies of the first edition were circulated over the world, mostly in the USA and Canada. Over 3000 of the readers have volunteered cooperation in the continuing studies. Not only is the Diet improving, curing and controlling a number of arthritic problems, but is revealing some recoveries from other diseases for which there are no known causes or controls. We hope to continue these survey studies for several years and also to seek funds for broadening the research efforts at interested institutions. For further information, see page 187.

To those who have secured a paperback copy, it would be appreciated if you would volunteer your help by reporting progress you may make (see last page of book) or any problems you may have solved or encountered. We are interested and shall try to give you assistance through the mail.

Most of the people who assisted so ably with the first edition of this book also have contributed to the second edition, plus thousands of additional cooperators. Miss Kim Doherty, a Cook College student of Rutgers University, has assisted with library and other studies. Dr. Joseph L. Evans and associates, Animal Nutrition, Cook College of Rutgers University, are conducting feeding experiments with rats to determine the effects of potato on movement of calcium and phosphorus in the blood system and body. This research is supported by the Wetterberg Foundation, Mr. Henry Parsons, Dayton, New Jersey. The assistance of all these people is appreciated very much.

The author will be happy to talk to interested groups about the Nightshades Diet for travel reimbursement and a modest fee.

January 1981 Norman F. Childers

Preface, First Edition

We should emphasize that material in this book is (a) largely background information on the economically important nightshade plants — the tomato, white potato, peppers, eggplant and smoking tobacco, and (b) a progress report on a lead to the cause and control of arthritic problems of humans. We are, indeed, humble about the impact this book could have on related commercial food, medical and drug industries. But is not human health uppermost?

We appear to have enough replies from over 400 of 600+ enrolled cooperators on the "No Nightshades" diet to make us reasonably sure we are on the track of something worth pursuing in human health. Like the cigarette-health situation, any adjustment in production and consumption of these botanically and chemically related crops likely would come slowly, if at all.

The nightshade food plants are very important and widely popular around the world. But people highly sensitive to the nightshades probably number less than ten percent of the population. Of course, there is a chance that the effects of the nightshade toxins could be subtle on humans and that it may take several decades to age and cripple people, some faster than others. In fact, we see few people from 70 to 90 years of age who do not have some form of stiffness or crippling that slows their movements. Considerable in-depth research is needed with the effects of these crops on man and animal covering several years.

We are almost certain that teams of medical scientists and agricultural food scientists working together can solve most of our nutritional health problems today if given the incentive and funds to do the job. We hope this book will help stir more interest in nutritional research for humans. Unfortunately, most of the curricula in medical colleges have not included training in plant, animal and human nutrition. The teaching and research effort has centered mainly on the development and use of new drugs, new technology in surgery, in psychiatry and other approaches to treat mostly the symptoms of diseases rather than to seek basic nutritional causes.

Agricultural scientists always have stressed the importance of nutritional work with both animals and plants. It is well known that if the plant has a nutritional problem, the animal eating that plant likely will have a problem, and the human eating the plant or animal or both eventually will develop a problem. It is generally recognized that the American farmer with the help of the Land Grant agricultural colleges has attained the highest production of quality food found anywhere in the world. We believe this same goal can be attained in good health and long life in humans if agriculturists can team up with the medical researchers in well funded, carefully planned projects.

Arthritis is an age-old disease, going back to dinosaurs millions of years ago. Their bones show the typical damage. Could they have fed on nightshades in the pastures? Today, it is interesting to note that carefully-fed livestock in America as horses and cattle usually die with all their teeth and with a skeletal system showing little if any deterioration. In fact, dairymen have metal caps placed on the worn teeth of cattle to extend their useful life in milk production. Why do humans experience dental and bone deterioration? Could there be abnormal movement of calcium and other minerals in the bones and blood system due to faulty nutrition? If it is nutrition, we are reasonably confident a medical-agricultural research team can solve it. We believe there is a good chance that cancer and heart diseases can be solved in the same manner.

We would like to thank the many friends who have helped us with this project and with the book. The encouragement "to do something about the diet-lead on arthritis" is much appreciated from Margery Stephenson, Charlotte Shafnacker, Marion Savoca and others in the Department of Horticulture and Forestry at Rutgers University. Alma P. Hough of Somerset Press, Inc., Somerville, New Jersey, gave much more help and encouragement than we probably should have accepted in more ways than we can enumerate. Credit also is due C. Palmer Bateman, Jr., President of Somerset Press, for his interest and help and also for that of his able staff in getting this book published. And, certainly, we wish to thank the hundreds of willing cooperators who are continuing to try the Diet of "No Night-shades" and who keep us posted on developments.

We sincerely hope we have started something that will benefit all of us. Comments, suggestions are always welcome.

Norman F. Childers
and
Gerard M. Russo

October 1977

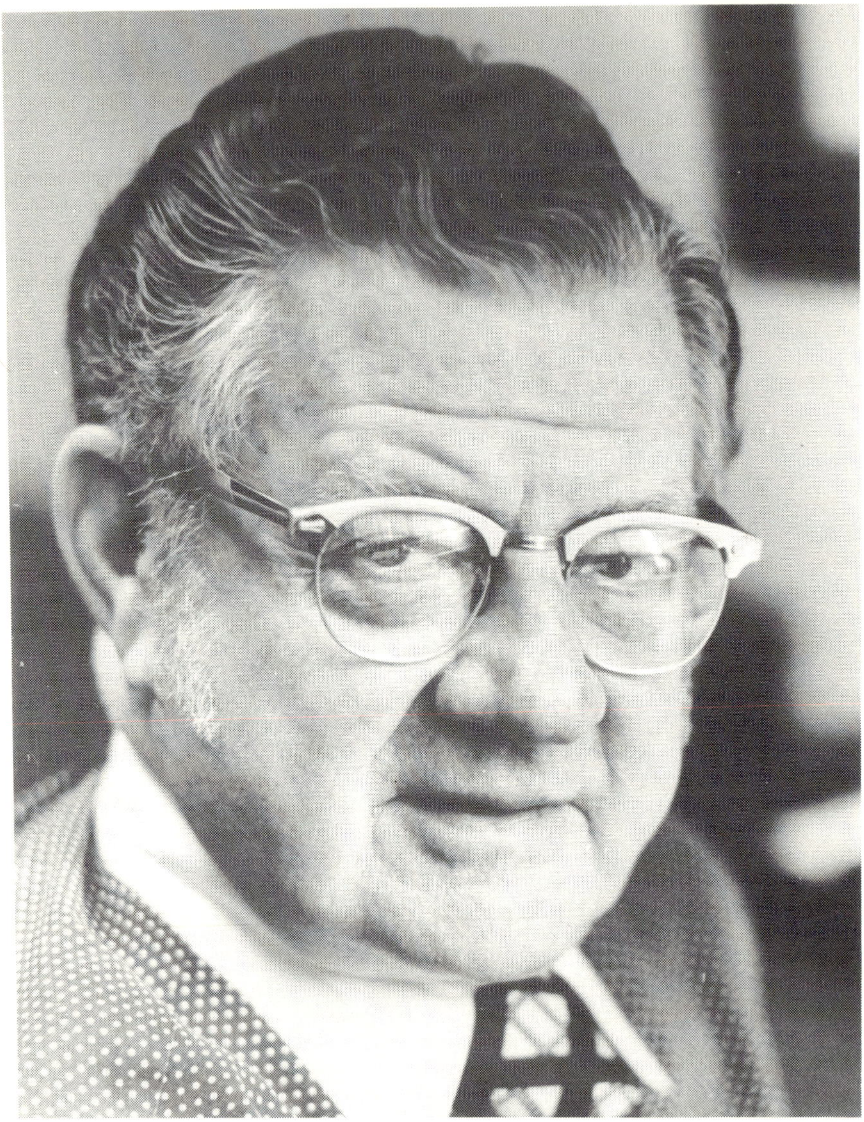

The Author, Dr. Norman F. Childers, is a graduate of the University of Missouri, Columbia, with a B.S. and M.S. degree, and of Cornell University, Ithaca, New York, with a PhD in Pomology and Plant Nutrition. He is Blake Professor of Horticulture, Cook College, Rutgers University, New Brunswick, New Jersey. (By F. A. Meyer, Philadelphia Evening Bulletin)

CHAPTER I

Introduction

It may sound overly optimistic to say that muscle stiffness, crippling, disability and the aches, pains and many discomforts of arthritis can be prevented, reduced or cured by controlling the diet and stopping the use of tobacco. *Total elimination of the nightshades* from daily usage by sensitive people (about 10% of the population) appears to be the important factor. The so-called nightshades include the *potato, tomato, tobacco, eggplant* and *all kinds of peppers* except the black pepper. There are a few other foods and factors that may be involved but the nightshades are the key.

By arthritis, the author is referring to musculoskeletal and connective tissue disorders as rheumatoid and osteoarthritis, bursitis, tennis elbow, gout, low back pain, anklyosing spondylitis, tendinitis, systemic lupus erythematosis and possibly a number of other related diseases. Response of cooperators in this study also indicates that neurological disorders as myasthenia gravis, multiple schlerosis, persistent headaches, depression and others could be related to consumption and usage of the nightshades. Certainly, these and other diseases should be checked. In fact, we would be glad to hear from and cooperate with anyone on the Diet who may be recovering from a disease for which the treatments have been ineffective. There are many of these diseases listed in the health manuals for which there is no known cause or control.[1]

Although we do not have adequate data at this time, there are indications from cooperators that heart attack (muscle spasm), hardening of the arteries, strokes, fast aging, high blood pressure, diverticulitis, kidney stones, breakdown of major organs and possibly cancer are related to the usage of the nightshades. Development of these diseases in the body is usually subtle and slow in coming. Arthritis appears to be only a symptom of the development of these other diseases. The National Institute of Health, Bethesda, Maryland, has noted that tobacco usage is related to several of the above diseases. The food nightshades are "first cousins" to tobacco. They all belong to the same plant family, the *Solanaceae.* It probably makes little difference whether the toxins of the nightshades enter the body and blood system through the lungs or through the alimentary canal.

Tobacco Correlates Easily

It is easy to correlate tobacco usage with human diseases. Smokers can be separated from non-smokers. But with the food nightshades everyone eats at least some of them almost every day. Based on experience in the

---

[1]The Merck Manual. 13th Ed. Merck, Sharp and Dohme Research Laboratories. Rahway, New Jersey. 2165 pp. 1977.

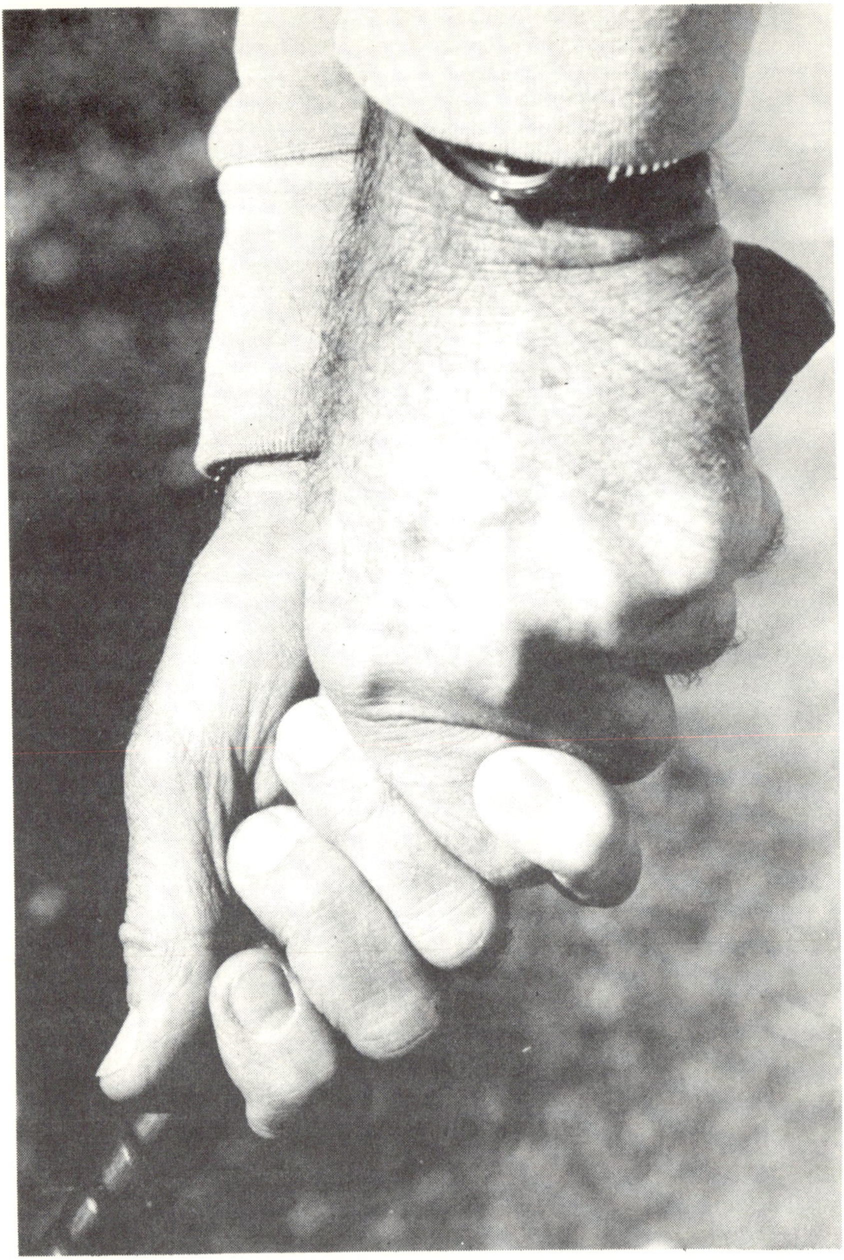

Figure 1. Nimble fingers, hands and arms, legs and back are paramount in many jobs. Many people are forced to retire or go to another job because of inability to handle a job physically. On the No-Nightshades Diet numerous cooperators have gone back to work and are "living a new life". Many improve their golf and sports! (Prof. Raymond P. Korbobo, Rutgers University, by Bob Costello, New Brunswick Home News.)

study reported here with thousands of arthritics over the world, mostly in the USA and Canada, at least 72% have improved or completely lost their aches, pains and swellings and some have discarded canes, walkers and wheelchairs, depending upon how far the disease has advanced. This is true only if the cooperators are able to avoid the nightshades *completely*. It is often said, "Once an arthritic, always an arthritic!" Arthritics generally appear to be highly sensitive to the nightshades and probably will continue to be sensitive as long as they live. They *must* adhere to this Diet to remain free of aches and pains and improve. These comments are based on 6 to 18 years of study discussed in this book.

In trying to do a diet, different people seem to proceed and react differently. Some find it a problem to do any diet, as e.g. losing weight. Attitude and sincerity are important. If a person hurts badly enough, however, he will do almost anything to get rid of his misery, even to the point of *completely* avoiding the nightshades, which it takes to get results. Many of the nightshades are "hidden" in a wide variety of prepared foods and only bits are enough to keep the problems going. People who simply "love" the nightshades, cannot do without them, eat or use them heavily, apparently are addicted to them as with tobacco, usually are the ones who get the aches, pains and problems first and the worst. Many complain of discomfort during and after the summer season of home gardening and when fresh vegetables are available in quantity in the markets and on roadside stands.

All Get Arthritis Eventually

Age seems to make little difference in sensitivity to the nightshades. Our studies show babies and teenagers suffer the same as senior citizens. History has shown that almost everyone will develop some form of arthritis sooner or later, certainly if they live into their 50s to 80s. As we have watched cooperators locally and listened to them by phone and in writing, it is not uncommon to find retired people who are on the Diet, eventually performing as they did in their 20s and 30s. In other words you may be able to add 10 to 20 years or more to your life. And these should be enjoyable years since you should regain agility, think and react faster and have a happy outlook with increased energy and endurance. Some Dieters have gone back to work after retirement. Some have gone back to school.

Again, this may sound overly optimistic, but thousands of cooperators have been receiving the benefits outlined above. Study the letters and case histories in Chapter III. You may identify with some of them.

The biggest deficiency in human health today is in nutrition and diet research. Advertising, media "news" and promotion sometimes have been misleading. Representative Margaret Heckler of Massachusetts, a member of the House Agricultural Committee, Washington, D.C., commented after a weekend on a Kansas farm, "There is more sophisticated dietary knowledge in the production of beef than there is in the medical profession

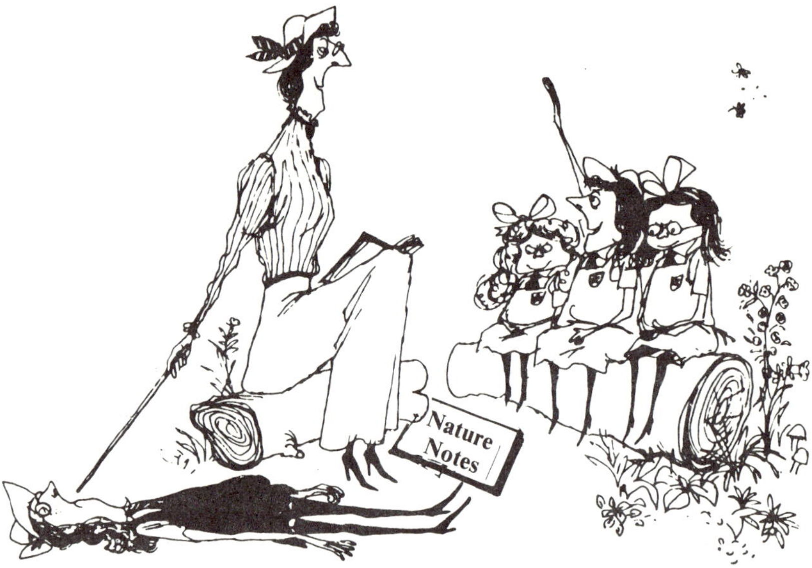

"Well done, Cynthia — it *WAS* deadly nightshade."

Figure 2. One needs only to go back 100s of years to find in old books and encyclopedias that people knew then the poisonous nature of the nightshade plants. They were reluctant to accept the potato and eggplant in Europe at first. Some are still skeptical of the tomato, calling it "The Cancer Apple". They called the eggplant "The Mad Apple" and tobacco, "The Dirty Weed"! This sketch was done by a Mr. Searle for *Lippiput* magazine in 1941 in Scotland. (Work Publishing Company, New York, N.Y.)

in the treatment of its patients". You will find this to be true not only in beef production but in all USA agriculture, covering both plants and animals. This is attributed to the missionary-like teaching and research in the agricultural colleges and experiment stations the past century.

This book is presented to you in all humbleness inasmuch as the author has been a professional horticulturist most of his life in university and experiment station research and teaching. His mission has been to try to show people how to grow better nightshades and other vegetables and fruits. But the "bottom line" really is our health and longevity! Obviously, there will be an impact of this book on the food, drug and the medical professions and industries, but it probably will be only moderate at most, as the case has been with the tobacco-health situation the past half-century.

Background

The nightshade plants *(Solanaceae* species) and their products long have been suspect in animal and human nutrition. Some are highly poisonous as the black and deadly nightshades *(Solanum nigrum* L. and *Atropa belladonna,* L. resp.). There are numerous beautiful ornamentals in the *Solanaceae* as petunia, chalice vine, day jessamine, and the Angel's and Devil's trumpet. Some have provided important medicinal drugs as belladonna, atropine and scopolamine, the latter being used widely in sleeping pills. Several are among our top food plants, as the tomato, white potato[1], garden peppers and the eggplant. Tobacco, also a closely related nightshade, known as "The Divine Plant" and "The Dirty Weed," has a questionable record in human health with respect to cancer, lung and heart diseases. There are some 90 genera in the *Solanaceae* family with over 2000 species[2]. The family ranks close to the grasses and legumes in importance to mankind.

Origin of the name, "Nightshade", is not clear. The English apparently called members of the *Solanum* genus, "Nightshades" because of their "evil and loving" narcotic nature of the night. Also the Latin word, *"solamen"* means quieting with sedative qualities. The Romans in the old days were said to prepare potions of the deadly nightshades and offer them to their enemies — the shade came down for a long night!

The White Potato. Charles B. Heiser, Jr.[3], of Indiana University, Bloomington, noted that the white potato, *Solanum tuberosum,* L. is called the "Earth's Apples". It comes from the highlands of Peru. The potato has been a staple food for centuries, especially for the Irish, providing high

---

[1]Strong, F.M. et al. Toxicants occurring naturally in foods. Nat. Acad. Sci., Second Ed. 624 pp. 1973.

[2]Bailey Horticultural Staff. Hortus Third. Macmillan Co., New York, N.Y. p. 1053. 1976.

[3]Heiser, C. B., Jr., Nightshades — The Paradoxical Plants. W. H. Freeman Co., San Francisco, Ca. 94101. 200 pp. 1969. This book gives interesting reading of the history, nature, and importance of the nightshades.

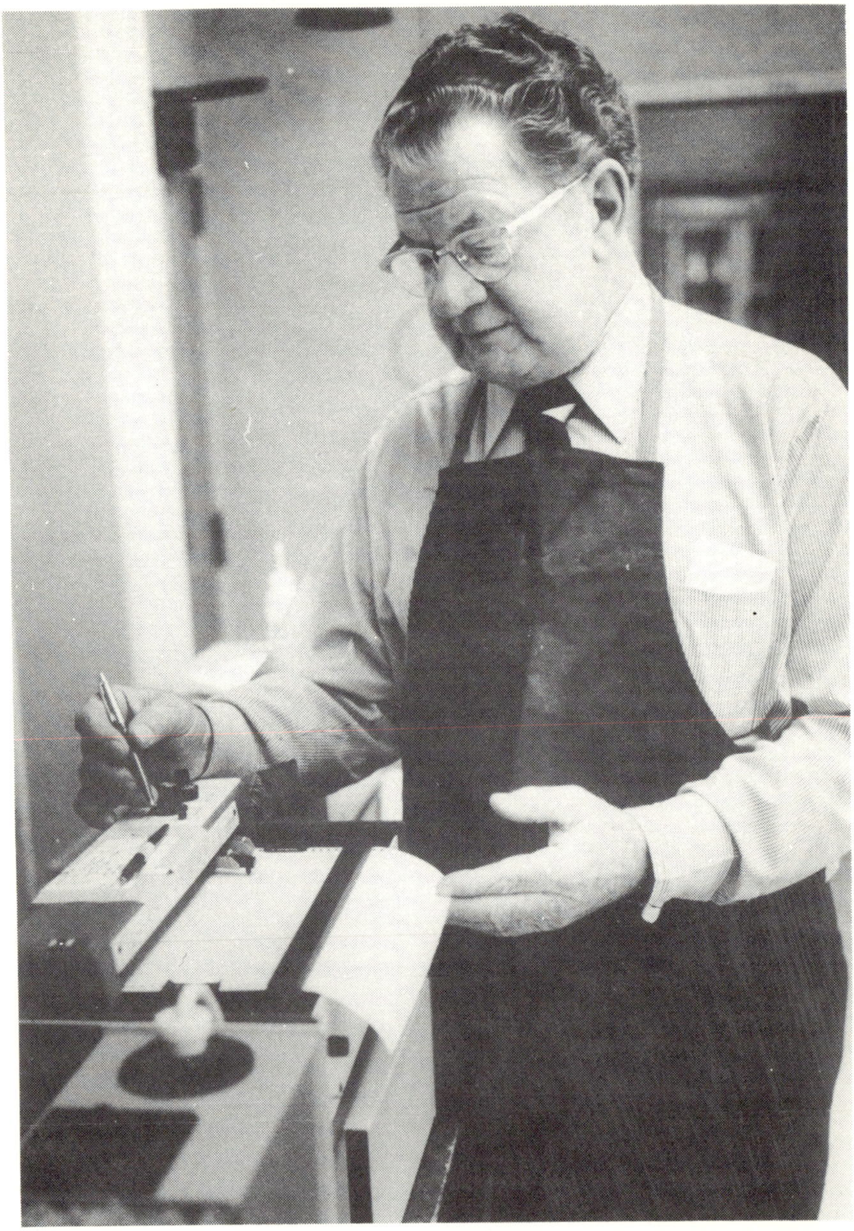

Toxins in the nightshade plants — the tomato, potato, eggplant, tobacco and peppers (except black pepper) — appear to have similar adverse effects on the health of both animals and man. Over 4500 different chemicals have been identified in tobacco with new ones being pin-pointed every year. Many toxins have been identified in the food nightshades but more research is needed in this area. (Photo by F.A. Meyer, Philadelphia Evening Bulletin).

food value and one of the few crops producing abundantly in their climate. During a famine in 1782, Scottish Highlanders complained of more than the usual dropsy (accumulation of fluid in joints) when potatoes were eaten abundantly due to shortage of other food[4].

The white potato contains the glycoalkaloid, *solanine,* among others, which is present throughout the potato but mostly in the peel. Solanine if ingested above the "safe level"[5] will cause toxic reactions in humans and animals, particularly if the potatoes are not selected, grown and handled properly (Zitnak's Chap.IV). Potato breeders have attempted to keep the solanine content of commercial potato cultivars below about 20 mg/100 gms fresh tuber[5]. It is thought that this content should be "safe" for human consumption. The potency of solanine can be appreciated when it is noted that if all the solanine (10,000 mgms) in 120 lbs of potatoes (av. U.S. per capita consumption) were fed to a horse at once, it would kill him.[6] Agricultural and medical researchers have been concerned with the solanine content of the white potato for decades, as noted in subsequent chapters. Solanine is not water soluble, is stable and is difficult to destroy by cooking.

Solanine is a powerful cholinesterase inhibitor. Cholinesterase is an enzyme in the body that affords agility of movement of the muscles. This may account for the stiffness and slow movement of some people susceptible to this inhibition. Humans may be divided roughly into three groups: (1) those fairly resistant to cholinesterase inhibition, (2) those moderately susceptible, and (3) those highly susceptible[7]. Kingsbury[8], Cornell Univ., says, "To associate this (cholinesterase inhibition) with the mechanism by which solanaceous alkaloids are toxic is an intriging thought begging experimentation."

A leading pest of the white potato and relatives is the Colorado potato beetle which seems to have a resistance to solanine glycoalkaloids and the cholinesterase-inhibiting type insecticides as Sevin. Hence, to control the beetle on potato plants, another type of insecticide had to be sought by entomologists. Many insect pests, can be controlled by cholinesterase-inhibiting compounds as nicotine in tobacco which causes spasms and paralysis in the insects. Livestock have died with some frequency in North America and Europe after ingesting potato vines, sprouts, peelings, and greened or spoiled potatoes. Human fatalities are documented. For a

---

[4]Salaman, R. History and Social influence of the potato. Cambridge University Press, Cambridge, England. 684 pp. 1949.

[5]Smith, Ora. Potatoes: Production, Storing, Processing, Avi. Publ. Co., Westport, Conn. Solanine. 94-6. 1968.

[6]Rpt. of Institute of Food Technologists, 221 No. LaSalle St., Chicago, Ill. 60601. March 1975.

[7]Orgell, W. H. et al. Inhibition of human plasma cholinesterase in vitro by extracts of *Solanaceae* plants. Science 128. 1136. 1958.

[8]Kingsbury, John M. Poisonous plants of the United States and Canada. Prentice-Hall, Englewood Cliffs, New Jersey. p. 288. 626 pp. 1968.

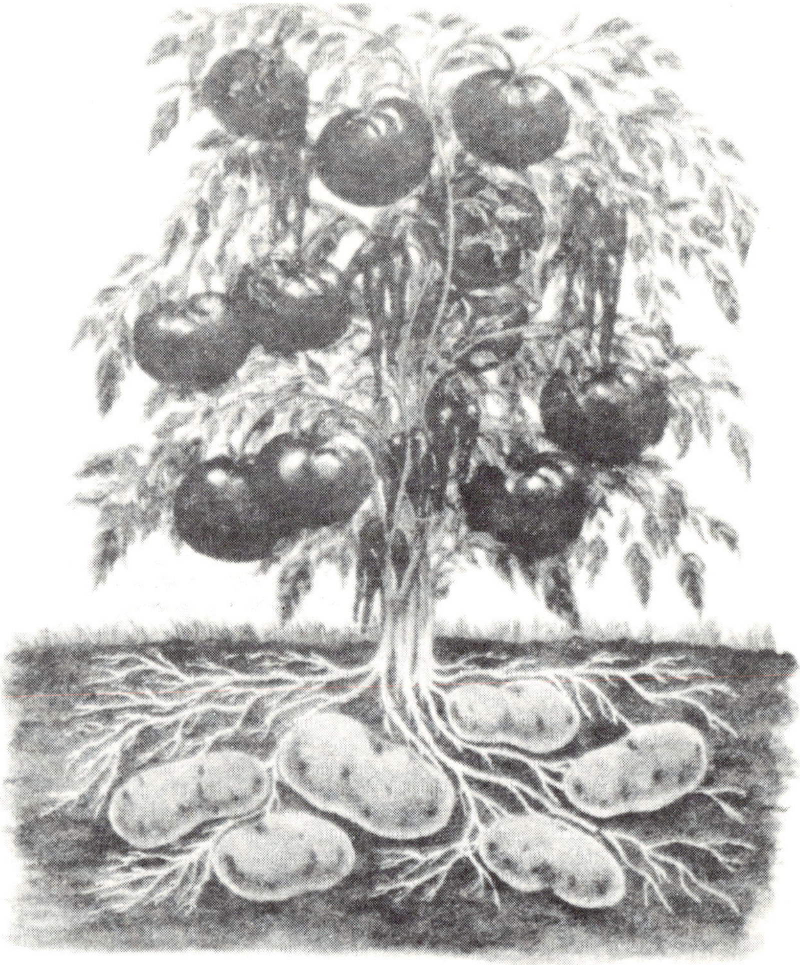

Figure 3. The tomato and pepper can be grafted onto the potato as indicated here. One nursery in Hanover, Pennsylvania is advertising the plant as a "Topeperatoe" (Toe-pep-er-atoe) in their catalogue. This indicates the close relationship of these crops with one another in the Nightshade *(Solanaceae)* family of plants. Tobacco and eggplant also can be intergrafted on these crops with various degrees of success.

Plants are grouped taxonomically by botanists on the basis of similarity of their flowers and fruits, primarily. Hence, a group of plants may have originated from a single plant, and variations have developed over the years by mutations.

detailed discussion of the poisonous nature of the nightshades and other plants, see the book by John M. Kingsbury[8].

Today, it is difficult to find a daily meal around the world without the white potato, prepared in one form or another. It ranks second to none in the production of calories per hectare. Over 90 percent of the world's crop is grown in Europe where it is used in much greater quantity for human and livestock food, for the production of alcohol, for the manufacture of synthetic rubber and for starch in sizing textiles and paper. In the United States it can be found in over 30 products on the grocery shelves. Potato flour or starch is used to give body to some breads, doughnuts, biscuits, candies, cookies and in soups. The potato is used in some baby foods. Odd to say, there was an old time remedy for arthritis of drinking the water in which potatoes had been boiled. Also, there was an old saying in New Hampshire shortly after the Irish brought the potato to the United States in 1719, that "white potatoes shortened men's lives"[9]

The Tomato. The tomato, *Lycopersicon esculentum,* L., is almost as important as the potato on world menus. Tomato production and consumption have grown tremendously in the USA since the early 1900s, are eaten fresh out-of-hand, in salads and processed into dozens of foods on the grocery shelves, including baby foods. The tomato is high in vitamins and low in starch whereas the potato is the opposite — low in vitamins and high in starch. The tomato and potato are closely related. The tomato apparently originated in the Peru-Ecuador-Bolivia area of the Andes[10] and was eaten by the American Indians long before it was taken to Europe and Africa, then returned to North America around the early 1900s. The tomato was termed "The Love Apple" and grown at first only as an ornamental. It was considered poisonous and disease producing and still is by some Europeans. The vines and suckers are poisonous to lifestock. Steroid alkaloids of the solanine type have been isolated from the tomato and other nightshades. (See Kingsbury's book). In olden times the tomato was referred to as the "The Cancer Apple"[11]. Polish literature shows that tomatine in the tomato has toxicity similar to solanine in the potato.

The tomato is now the No. 1 processed food in the USA due to heavy usage in fast-food restaurants as tomato sauce and other products, which have moved from 9 lbs/capita in 1965 to over 15 lbs in the late 1970s.

The Green Pepper. The garden pepper includes *Capsicum frutescens,* L. which according to Hortus Third[12] is the Tobasco pepper; and *C. Annuum* L. which is the cherry, red cluster, bell, sweet, green, pimiento, chili, long and red peppers. The garden pepper should not be confused with the

---

[9]Scott, J. D. Praise The Potato! Reader's Digest. New York. p. 206, December 1976.
[10]The World in Your Garden. National Geographic Soc., Washington, D.C. 112-13. 1957.
[11]Early American Horticulture. Grower Talks. Bicentenial Issue. George J. Ball, Inc. West Chicago, Illinois. p. 48. July 1976.
[12]Bailey Hortorium Staff. Hortus Third. The Macmillan Co., New York. p. 219. 1290 pp. 1976.

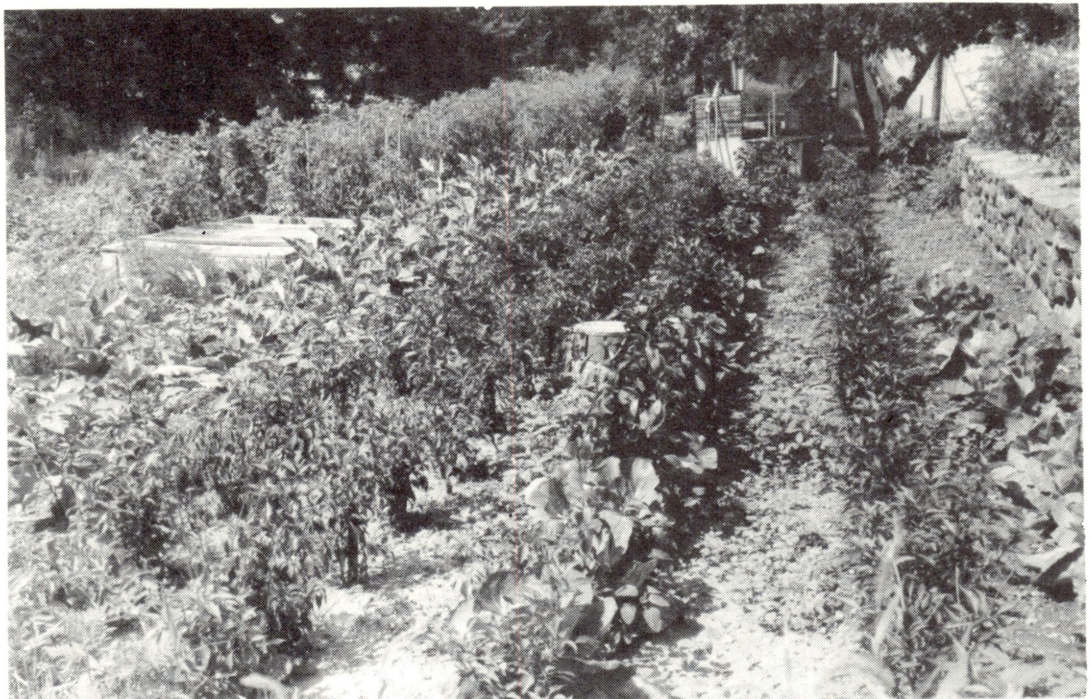

Figure 4. For people sensitive to nightshades, the aches and pains of arthritis seem to intensify during the summer home garden and roadside market season. Above is a typical garden with many nightshades. They are easy to grow, productive and delectable. From left to right: Tomatoes in rear, eggplants, sweet green and red peppers in the cabbage row, and skinny hot peppers on the far right.

black or condiment pepper which is a small berry of a tropical vine, *Piper nigrum* L. of the *Piperaceae* family, *not* the *Solanaceae* family. Black pepper does not aggravate arthritis.

Paprika, which is found in many items on the grocery shelves and sprinkled on seafoods and other dishes, comes from a long, thick, non-pungent pepper mostly grown in Hungary. The USA imports of this pepper approach 6000 metric tons a year; California produces about 7000 metric tons. The Tobasco pepper is the basis of the pungent Tobasco sauces made in Louisiana and used widely around the world. The cayenne pepper is the dried ground fruit of a long slender hot pepper named after a coastal city in French Guiana. Pimento, or pimiento, peppers are the mild sweet kinds in Spain or the thick-fleshed bright red sweet peppers in the United States, used to decorate salad dishes, in olives and cut into bits in rice, peas, shelled corn, etc. Chili (from Chili) peppers in Spain are the hot kinds, as in the United States, and used, e.g., in chili con carni.

The garden peppers also originated in Peru, having been found in the embroidery on an Indian garment in Peruvian ruins, used there more than 2000 years ago. Mexicans today eat incredible quantities of hot peppers of the fresh green and red ripe, dried mature forms. The hot red pepper is widely used in many foods throughout the southern United States. Hot pepper also is used in the tropics to mask off-flavor meat that has not been refrigerated properly, if at all. Hot pepper may cause skin rash to people harvesting and handling the crop. Mailmen have used spray potions to repel dogs and a preparation is used to stop babies from sucking their thumbs. For some people it can cause an inflamed alimentary canal and serious digestive problems.

There is a wealth of information on the chemical composition of the pepper, as noted in Dr. Zitnak's Chapter IV.

The Eggplant. The eggplant, *Solanum Melongena,* L. also was grown as an ornamental in the early days and was not widely eaten until relatively recent years. In the Mediterranean area it was thought to cause insanity if eaten daily for a month. In fact, it was called "The Mad Apple" which may have come from the Italian name, *melazana,* or the pre-Linnean name, *Mala insana.* The eggplant is thought to have originated in the Assam/Burma area of India. It was introduced into American gardens in 1806 as an ornamental, then grown for food only in the present century. Some cultivars grown under certain conditions may develop considerable bitterness, probably due to the high solanine content in the skin area. There is little information on the chemical composition of the eggplant. There are dozens of shapes, sizes and kinds of fruits ranging from small round to long banana-like, and colored from white to red, orange, ashen, purple, brown and black. General consumption of the eggplant is much less than the other nightshades.

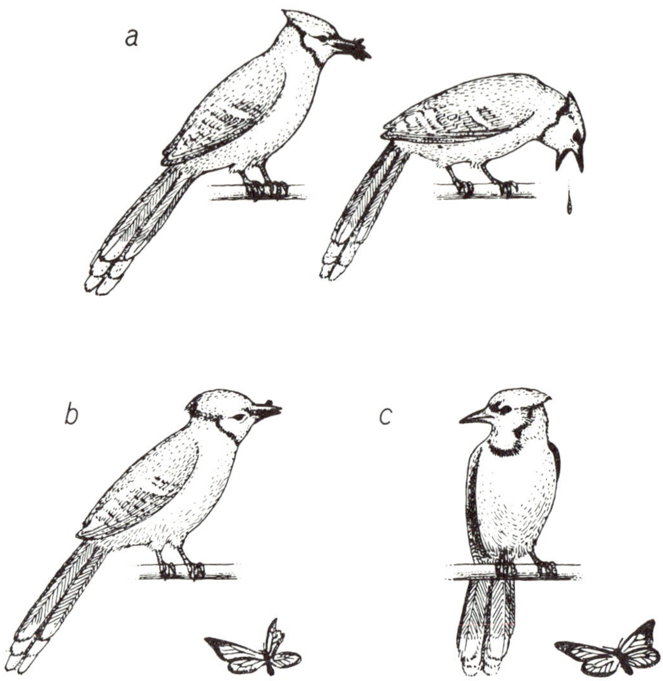

Figure 5. Are we as aware as birds, animals? A colt may eat a nightshade weed unknowingly in the pasture and die before its mare can "warn" it. If birds ingest poisonous matter, they vomit, learn their lesson and shy away from that food thereafter. Above, (a) when a bird, or blue jay in this instance, is made ill by an insect, it vomits, then associates the flavor of the insect with the illness and thereafter will reject an insect by tasting it (b). Tests were made by Dr. L. P. Brower, Amherst College, Mass., with monarch butterflies that had or had not eaten leaves of the poisonous milkweed in the larval stage. At (c) birds usually learn to reject such insects on sight. Chemicals in the poisonous milkweed are classified as "cardiac glycosides". (Readings from Scientific American, W. H. Freeman & Company, San Francisco. No. 15. 134-162. 1973.)

Other Solanaceous Crops. Mention should be made of the husk tomato, or "ground cherry" *(Physalis pubescens,* L) which is grown in many home gardens but not commercially. One of our cooperators in Kentucky kept complaining of sore inflamed hands until we identified the "ground cherry" as a member of the *Solanaceae* family. The garden huckleberry *(Solanum nigrum,* L) has leaves and berries that should be avoided by arthritics. It also is known as Morelle, wonderberry and sunberry. The cherry and plum tomatoes often served in restaurants are genetic variations of the common larger tomatoes, as is true also of yellow tomatoes. All aggravate arthritics.

Other "edible" solanaceous crops include the pepino *(Solanum muricatum,* Ait.), European bitter sweet *(Solanum Dulcamara,* L.), tree tomato *(Cyphomandra betacea,* Senot.), tomatillo *(Physalis ixocarpa,* Brot.), strawberry tomato *(Physalis prinosa,* L.) and Cape gooseberry (*P. peruviana,* L.). All of these crops, leaves or fruit, likely will cause arthritics problems.

Home Gardens. The nightshade food plants are easy to grow in home gardens and are highly favored because of their delectable products and productiveness in a limited space. Many susceptible people who have home gardens seem to develop aches and pains in their backs, wrists, hands, shoulders, elbows, chests and/or hips in late summer after they have eaten voraciously of the nightshades from their home gardens and the roadside markets. Many cooperators have reported skin rash, headaches, asthma and other minor health problems after woi king with the nightshades in the garden, the market or processing plant.

Within the past few decades the American diet has tilted heavily toward the nightshades. Where in former years we ate mostly mashed potatoes patty cakes, or boiled potatoes with the skins removed, now we have baked potatoes (skins are high in solanine), or French fries with ketchup. Now we eat pizzas, ketchup on many things, and salads almost daily (from the salad bar) with fresh tomatoes and peppers. Tomato juice for breakfast, as an appetizer, in "Bloody Mary's", or as a good cold drink any time of day has become quite common. Fast food restaurants use enormous quantities of the nightshade foods, which could account for much of the ill effects of so-called "Junk Foods" on mainly the younger generation.

Symptoms of Nightshade Poisoning. John M. Kingsbury (his book noted under white potato) makes the interesting statement that, "Despite the ancient and general reputation of nightshades as poisonous plants, very few feeding experiments have been performed with any of the toxic species. It is generally believed that toxicity of a given species may vary over wide limits with factors of its environment, part of plant, and degree of maturity. Genetics may play a part."

The symptoms and lesions caused by the many species of *Solanum* and relatives are quite uniform even though their chemical composition is somewhat different. The saponic-like glycoalkaloid is an irritant and in physical characteristics causes red blood cell destruction *in vitro*. The steroid alkamine is readily absorbed by the intestine and responsible for the nervous symptoms. Responses in animal and man are similar.

Gastrointestinal irritation: This may be either slight or severe enough to overshadow nervous effects. Includes anorexia (loss of appetite), nausea (dizziness), abdominal pain, vomiting, constipation or diarrhea (sometimes with blood), red blood cell loss, wasting, rough wrinkled skin, skin rash, jaundice, and accumulation of fluid in abdomen tissue. Results in lesions in animals (ulcers or diverticulitis in humans?) which vary from minor inflammation of the mucosae to ulceration and hemmorrhage. Lesions accounting for the nervous symptoms have not been found. Symptoms and lesions are comparable in the human being and various classes of livestock. Acute poisoning is almost always involved and follows the course described below. Occasionally, chronic poisoning occurs. This happened in Canada in recent years when vegetable researchers ate a quantity of the 'Lenape' cultivar of potato found later to be high in solanine content. They developed the usual symptoms, and the variety was quickly withdrawn and placed under number for future breeding purposes (since it was of high yield and solids content, making excellent potato chips).

Nervous effects: Includes apathy, drowsiness, salivation, dyspnea (difficult breathing), trembling, progressive weakness, paralysis, prostration and eventual unconsciousness. (Pupil dilation is not diagnostic of solanine poisoning.) In humans the symptoms of stupefaction and loss of sensations are apparent. In acute poisoning nervous symptoms build to maximum, and death or recovery eventuates within a few hours to one or two days. Death is the result of paralysis (heart attack?). Solanine poisoning is not always fatal.

The National Problem of Pains

Cima Star in Family Weekly, March 6, 1977, noted that "Chronic pain . . . costs the society in the United States an estimated $50 billion a year in medical expenses, loss of wages and worker-compensation benefits." According to John J. Bonica, President of the International Association for the Study of pain, chronic back pain alone, the most common problem, disables seven million people annually and is responsible for nearly 19 million visits to doctors each year." Based on our cooperators' replies to omitting the nightshades from their diet, it appears that these crops play a major role in most of these back problems.

Verona L. Van Pelt, R. N., Lancaster, Virginia, has brought to our attention the following book written bv Alida Frances Pattee for nurses, "Practical Diatetics with Reference to Diet in Disease", 3rd Ed., 360 pp.,

1905, A. F. Pattee, Publisher, 52 W. 52nd St., NYC, in which she suggests *avoiding tomato and potato to control aches and pains of "rheumatism"*, the word used in olden days instead of "arthritis".

Interesting Relationships

The Chinese eat mostly rice, grain and soybeans in place of potatoes, very few tomatoes, but they produce and consume large quantities of eggplant and peppers in one form or another, particularly in South China. Tobacco is used widely. The Chinese have the major diseases found in the USA — heart attack, high blood pressure, arthritis and cancer. The Japanese in recent years have switched to some extent to an American-type diet that includes French fries, tomatoes, eggplant, pizzas, etc. Stomach cancer and heart diseases are increasing among the Japanese who eat also pickled foods some of which include the nightshades.

The late Dr. C.H. Dong[13], Chinese born in California, spent time in China, studied medicine, received his MD degree from the Stanford Medical School in California, tells the story of how he developed a serious case of arthritis after switching to the American diet, and eventually developing a special diet with Jane Banks, co-author, and the cooperation of hundreds of his patients. They frown upon tomatoes and peppers in any form including spices, among other things. He concludes that, "My dramatic recovery convinces me that rheumatic diseases are caused by chemical poisoning put into our food . . . . and by allergy to certain foods." Thus, he contends the basis for arthritis is in the human diet. Dr. Myron Rosenbaum MD, in a recent book[14] also concludes that diet is likely involved in arthritis, but he is unable to pinpoint the culprits.

The Irish who serve potatoes with most daily meals and the Mediterranean peoples who use an abundance of tomatoes, peppers and eggplant are plagued with a high percentage of arthritis and other key diseases. Our cooperator files are heavy with these ethnic groups and they usually have great difficulty adapting to a diet omitting these foods.

The Eskimos who have eaten largely meat until recent years are less bothered with the major health diseases found in America and Europe. They have had little or no arthritis, cancer or heart attacks. The Hunzas[15] in the Himalayas above India do not have a cancer problem[15] and they are said to live to 100-150 years. There may be other correlations with ethnic groups and disease problems. An in-depth study of these groups and others could be highly fruitful.

---

[13]Dong, Collin H. and Jane Banks. New Hope For The Arthritic. Thomas H. Crowell Co., New York, N.Y. 269 pp. 1975.

[14]Rosenbaum, Myron G., MD. Understanding Arthritis. W. H. Green, Inc., St. Louis, Mo., 63105, 102 pp. 1979.

[15]Peeters, Emile-Gaston and Yola Verhasselt, Impact, Publ. by UNESCO, Paris, France. (Research at Vrije University of Brussells, Belgium.)

The Arthritic Lead

The author of this book over 18 years has been studying personal aches and pains, starting with diverticulitis and the 3-phase operations with a colostomy. The local surgeon, Rudolph Matflerd, MD, indicated possibly spices as the cause, or "hot" foods. In tracing back, the only difference in daily routine that could have aggravated diverticulitis was heavy consumption of a spiced tomato juice which was causing a tingling of the legs, difficulty in getting oriented in bed at night, and in sleeping. Later, fresh tomatoes or tomatoes in any form were found to cause soreness in joints and muscles within an hour or two after eating them. Then the innocent white potato was pinpointed, followed by the pepper and the eggplant which had considerable clout. Being a horticulturist, it is well known to us that these food crops are closely related, including smoking tobacco.

The survey-test. The effects of the nightshades on the author were mentioned to friends who had similar problems and they, in turn, tried the "No-Nightshades" Diet with similar results. They urged the author "to do something about it" to help other people. Hence, with a few small ads in limited circulation news media, and numerous items about the Diet discussed subsequently in the media, we assembled some 3000 cooperators at this writing in about 6 years. We have heard from about 30+ % of these cooperators during the past year. The data are given in Table 1 below. Most cooperators have had some degree of improvement, some complete relief and some reporting marked improvement.

Table 1. Response of cooperators to the "No-Nightshades" diet-survey conducted August 1979.

Response Description	Number Cooperators	Number Practiced Diet: Rigidly	Somewhat	Not	Percent Of Total
Marked Positive[1] Response	216*	178	38	0	28.3
Positive Response[2]	340	183	157	0	44.4
Not On Diet[3]	151	8	56	87	19.8
Negative Response[4]	56	24	9	23	7.5
Totals	763	393	260	110	100.0

[1]Marked, "unbelievable" improvement; discarding wheelchairs, walkers, canes; immobile joints now mobile or becoming mobile.

[2]Noticeable response, many still with problems.

[3]Comments indicate not actually on diet, as "Cannot resist tomatoes on occasion", "These staples too difficult to avoid."

[4]Apparently tried diet, 40% rigidly, for several weeks or months or a year or more without improvement. But 55% said they are still on the diet, more or less.

*These cooperators have been on the diet 6 months or more, some 3½ yrs.

In August 1979, questionnaires were sent to about 2400 cooperators requesting a quick reply on a stamped return card so the author could present the data at a meeting of the International Academy of Preventative Medicine in St. Louis, Missouri in September. You will note in Table 1 that replies were received from 763 cooperators in this short time. Of the 763 replies, 556 were getting positive results or about 72%. When the cooperators were on the Diet "Rigidly", more were getting positive results and better results than those "Somewhat" on the Diet. You will note that some of those on the Diet were discarding canes, walkers and wheelchairs.

The question always arises as to what happened to those who did not reply. There could be many reasons. Some move to another address, some have passed away, and others are just not good correspondents, at least for a quick reply. Some may have become discouraged because of slow, if any, response to the Diet. And this could be due to many factors, as over-medication, excess use of vitamin and supplement pills, over-shadowing of another disease, not really wanting to give up the nightshades, did not want their identity revealed, and, perhaps most important, did not really understand the diet, and saying they are on the Diet when actually they are not.

The response we got to the questionnaire is fairly good which was over 30%. In any case, there is an indication that quite a number of people are responding to the Diet and it should be of interest to arthritics, particularly those who have had the problem for many years and have tried almost "everything" with little or no success. It should be noted that where we can work with cooperators locally and check with them periodically to help perfect the Diet, the cooperators nearly always get strong positive results.

Where the Diet has helped most. Young people with little or no bone, joint or tendon damage seem to benefit quickly on the Diet when their aches and pains are beginning to develop. Middle-age people (40s to 60s), likewise may be relieved of their aches and pains if the problem has been with them only a few years. However, if there is bone and vertebrae damage, some fusion and pressure on nerves, then one can expect 9 to 12 months, maybe longer, strictly on the Diet before improvements may start. Generally, the problem does not worsen and usually there is improvement if the person has the patience to stay with the Diet faithfully. In most arthritics there is very gradual improvement over as much as 6 years, the extent of our tests thus far. How far noticeable disfigurement can improve with time, one cannot be sure, but there undoubtedly is a limit. Surgery may be in order to relieve pressure on nerves and where there is damage to the skeletal system. Then continue the Diet permanently to avoid further damage.

With more time and more cooperators, we should be able to make a better and clearer long-term evaluation. It appears to us that we have one of the better answers to the cause and control of arthritic/rheumatic aches and pains and associated health deterioration. Most cooperators have proven to themselves the effectiveness of the Diet by avoiding the nightshades for 3 to 6 months, then going off the Diet for a week or two to find the aches and pains returning and/or intensifying. Success of the Diet seems to lie in one's ability to stay away from the nightshades *completely* during the test period, avoid over-medication and excessive use of vitamins and supplements. In fact, in most cases, the latter three items should be gradually reduced and stopped, or taken only intermittently if testing has developed problems or shown no good reason for taking them. For those people susceptible to the nightshades, apparently they must reconcile themselves to permanent abstinence from them, or reap the consequences.

People who use tobacco, particularly cigarette smokers, are usually indifferent about the Diet at first, mainly because of their known difficulty in trying to stop the habit. The few cooperators who have been able to stop cigarettes while on the Diet, find a return of low-key aches and pains when they go back to smoking, but less intense than when they also were partaking of the nightshade foods.

Health Improvements Associated With The Diet: Several ailments or problems that have been improved or corrected by the Diet for cooperators include:

Inflamed, swelling of the knees, feet and hands.
Skin rash.
Thinning of the blood.
Tennis elbow.
Tender nipples of men.
Chest pains as if man were standing on it.
Pelvic aches, pains.
Sluggish mind, body, muscles in general.
Mental depression.
Lack of ambition and desire to do things.
Reduced calcium on teeth.
Eliminated Fever Blisters.
Poor endurance.
Ups and downs from day to day in attitude as feeling good or bad.
Bleeding from lower colon.
Fading liver spots.
Reduced size of moles, warts.
Less visits to the doctor, dentist, hospital.
Better eye sight and hearing.
Better awareness.
Loss of heart pains down left arm.
Correction of diverticulitis attacks if so troubled.
Reduced ulcer problems.
Clearing of aches and pains in muscles and joints.
Reduction in or no more headaches.
Loss of diarrhea attacks.
Better sleep and rest.
Calmer, more endurance.
More ambition.
Better outlook.
Better complexion.
Look younger, feel younger.
Better libido (probably due to better health).
Reduced or loss of muscle spasms in back and limbs (as a "charley horse" or "crick" in back).
Loss of "growth pains" in children.
Lowering of blood pressure to normal.

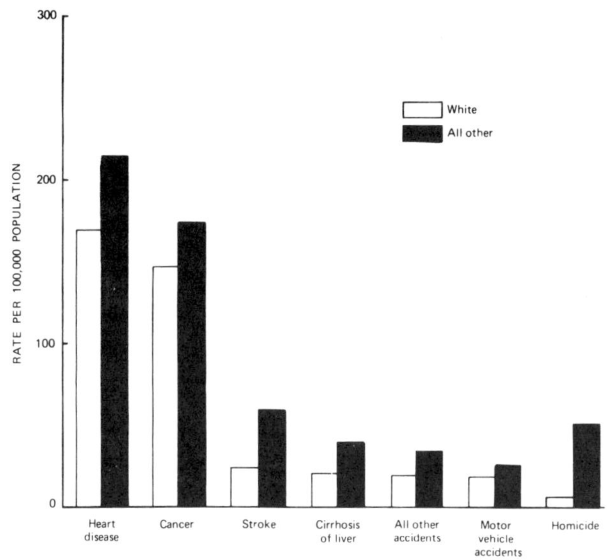

Figure 6. Chart shows the major causes for death of people 25-64 years of age in USA, 1976. Cardiovascular diseases and cancer lead. Cirrhosis of liver may be associated with alcoholism. (Nat. Cen. for Health Stat., U. S. Gov'n.)

The aches and pains of arthritis seem to settle in one location today and in another location tomorrow. They are attracted first to areas where there has been stress or tissue and bone damage, apparently due to the settling of the nightshade toxins, as solanine, near severed dead-end blood vessels. Vitamin D_3 in the nightshades, as indicated in Chapter VI, may be involved in the movement and deposits of calcium and phosphorus from the blood in the damaged areas. The aches and pains usually disappear last from those areas where the damage has been significant and of long standing.

The Nightshades and Other Diseases

Heart Attack. It is widely accepted that the tobacco nightshade is involved in heart attacks (Chap. V). It is conceivable that where a person may be eating rather heavily of tomatoes, potatoes, perhaps a pepper and an eggplant and/or smoking a pack or two of cigarettes a day, that a muscle spasm could result and settle in a limb or in the heart, causing a problem one day whereas there was no health problem the previous day. A characteristic of the nightshades under some conditions is to paralyze the muscles and nervous system. This is how the 40% nicotine sulphate

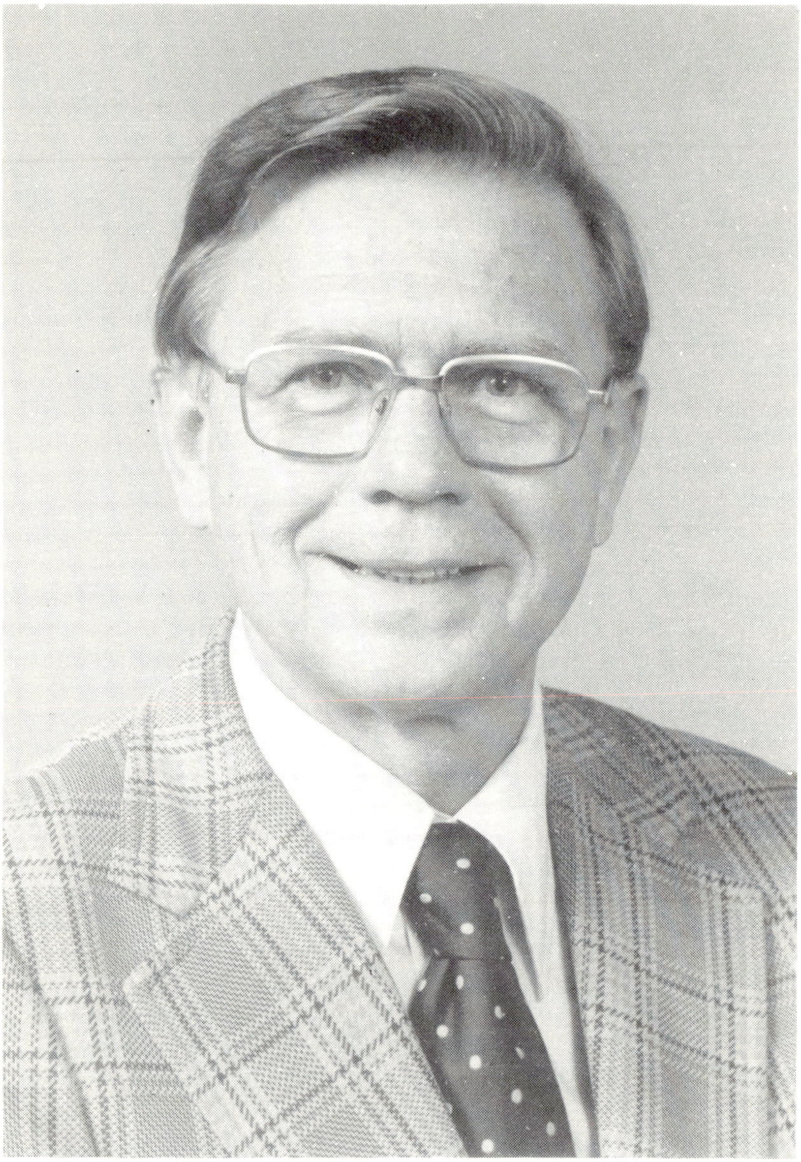

Albert A. Kattus, M.D., University of California at Los Angeles observed a muscle spasm during a cardiac by-pass operation, the cause unknown. He found the coronary artery to be "tough like twine and not soft and pliable". Use of the tobacco nightshade has been associated with heart attacks. Other nightshades can cause muscle paralysis and should be checked. This awareness of spasm is leading to a new line of attack against heart problems.

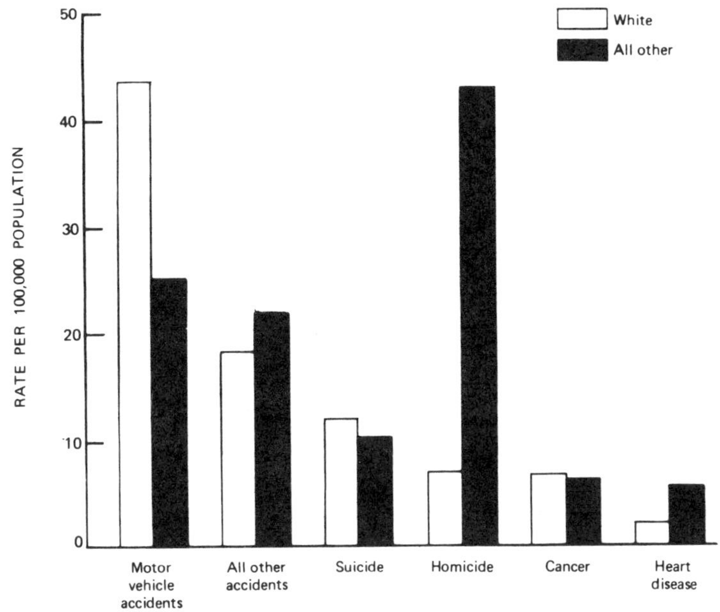

Figure 7. Chart shows major causes of death for young people, ages 15-24 years of age, 1976. Cancer and heart disease are lowest in rate per 100,000. (Nat. Cen. for Health Stat., U.S. Gov'n.)

pesticide from tobacco kills insects. This is how people have died (documented) or become seriously ill from eating the nightshades under certain conditions. Nicotine extracted from several cigars (in prison, e.g.) can be used to poison (heart attack) another person.

A recent item appearing in Time magazine (Nov. 26, 1979) carried the heading, "Spasm Causes Heart Attack". Medical doctors often assume that heart attacks are triggered by blood clots or atherosclerotic plaques clogging the arteries that supply oxygen-rich blood to the heart muscle. But in the case cited by Time, the heart blood vessels were checked and found free from clots. The theory of spasm in heart muscles dates back to the early 1900s but there has been no observed proof that a spasm causes a heart attack. Cardiologist Albert A. Kattus MD[16] of the University of California at Los Angeles has observed a heart spasm during a heart operation, cause unknown. Dr. Attilo Maseri while at the University of Pisa, Italy, worked with a significant number of patients with atherosclerosis and chest pains and found that they were due to spasms. While a spasm may only hinder the blood flow, a blockage could occur in vessels already narrowed by fatty deposits (see Chap. VI by Dr. Davis on Vitamin D_3 as a culprit). A spasm could be triggered by psychological stress, an over-worked heart needing rest, or a release of thromboxane A_2. Also, as indicated above, the chemicals in the nightshades such as nicotine in tobacco

[21]Kattus, A.A. Coronary artery spasm: new appraisal. Ann. Rev. Med. *27*:69-75.1976.

are known to cause blood vessel constriction and muscle paralysis. The food nightshades should be checked as a causal factor. According to Time, this awareness of muscle spasm is leading to a new line of attack against heart disease.

Note in Figure 6 that heart disease in the USA leads other diseases for people between the ages of 25 to 64 years. Note also that arthritis is not listed as a cause of death, or at least not important enough to include in this chart. Arthritis appears to be only a symptom of other diseases developing in the body that eventually result in death. Hence, one should acknowledge this symptom and proceed to reduce it or control it as early as possible. The nightshades apparently are the key factor involved in arthritis and could lead to other diseases. Note in Figure 7 that cancer and heart disease rank fifth and sixth, resp., for young people, 15-24 years.

Cancer. Again, the tobacco nightshade is widely recognized as a factor causing cancer, particularly in the respiratory channels (see Chap. IV by Dr. Tso). Figure 8, published in the first edition of this book, is of interest with respect to stomach cancer. The tomato, as pointed earlier in this Chapter, was called in early times "The cancer apple". Diverticulitis, which in the author's experience apparently was induced by excessive amounts of a spiced tomato juice (contains hot pepper), is often a precursor of bowel cancer. In persistent cases, medical advice is to remove the affected intestinal area by surgery. In people over 50 years of age, 30 to 40% are judged to have diverticula, often unknown to the individual, and the incidence increases with each subsequent decade of life. Bowel cancer is becoming a leading cause of death in middle-age and older people. Since the tobacco nightshade is associated with the development of cancer, it would seem wise to check also its close relatives, the food nightshades. It is interesting that (a) some moles (a cancer caution) gradually disappear on the Diet, and (b) Eskimos (who eat largely meat), and (c) Hunzas have little or no cancer.

The mortality rate for Iowa farmers from six kinds of cancer is much higher than for Iowa non-farmers, as reported by Dr. Leon Burmeister head of a project in preventative medicine and environmental health, University of Iowa, Iowa City (a media interview in April 1980). The study was based on 20,311 white Iowa farm men from 1971 to 1978, concluding that farmers were more likely to die from leukemia, prostatic, lip, stomach, bone marrow, and lymphatic cancers than non-farmers. Farmers, however, were less susceptible to tobacco-related cancers than urban people. The results were surprising since the general concept is that farmers are healthier than city people. Dr. Burmeister indicated that farmers may be more susceptible to certain kinds of cancer because of their proximity to animal viruses, farm chemicals and dust from hay and ensilage. Coming from the mid-west farming business, as the book author does (Missouri), we well know that most farmers have meat and potatoes three times a day for energy to carry

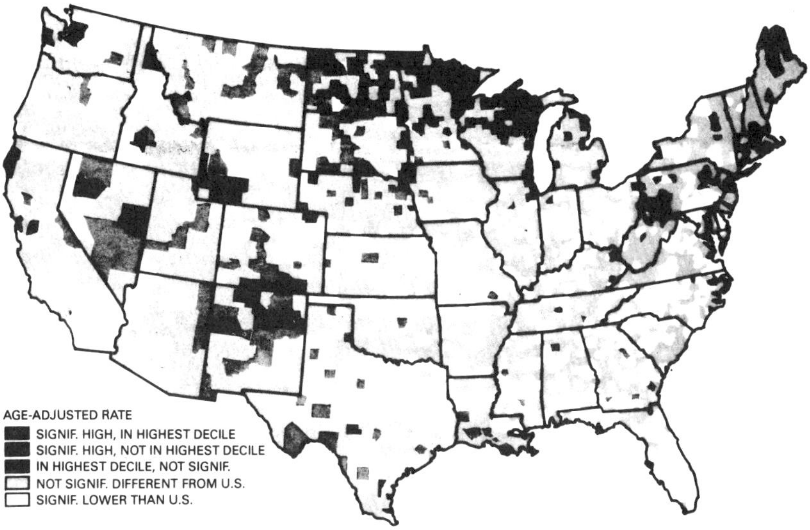

Figure 8. Chart shows stomach cancer mortality in white males by county, USA, 1950-69. R.S. Adams, Jr., University of Minnesota, notes that darker areas tend to be remote from urban centers where "natives are likely to rely more on their home gardens and often-untreated water supplies". Could nightshades play a part, since these crops often dominate in home gardens? Also, note that commercial potato production tends to fall in many of the black areas. In these areas, potatoes are readily available, not so expensive, and farmers may eat more. (From "Down To Earth", Dow Chem. Co., Midland, Mi. *32:*3.p. 6-13. Winter 1976; and Mason et al., Publ. No. NIH 75-780, USD Health, Educ., Welfare, 1975.)

on! They also have a ready supply of nightshade vegetables from their home gardens (Figure 3).

There is a question of *artificial sweeteners* and the incidence of bladder cancer. Drs. E. L. Wynder and S. D. Stellman[17], American Health Foundation, New York City, report a case-control study of 302 male and 65 female bladder cancer patients and an equal number of control patients matched with them in age, sex and hospital-room status. They found no association between use of artificial sweeteners or diet beverages and bladder cancer. No dose-response was observed with respect to quantity or duration of use of the two combined. No evidence was found that suggests artificial sweeteners or diet beverages promote the tumorigenic effect of tobacco smoking. In any case, it probably is wise to use saccharin moderately.

[17]Wynder, E. L. and S. D. Stellman. Artificial sweetener use and bladder cancer: a case-control study. Science 207: March 14, 1214-16. 1980.

In Summary. Our knowledge in human nutrition and of what is "the proper diet" is grossly inadequate in the world today. Anything you as readers can do to boost the nutritional research programs in both the food (agricultural) and medical professions will bring us answers that much sooner.

Agricultural Research And Human Health

The agricultural experiment stations over the country have been operating productively since and before the 1900s. They are well equipped with highly trained and dedicated staffs in the production of quality food. Working as a team with the medical researchers, we should be able to accelerate the solution of key human health problems associated with the diet. Cancer and cardiovascular diseases could fall into this classification and possibly alcoholism and drug addiction. There are dozens of other human diseases for which we have no answer as to cause.

Agricultural researchers are thoroughly acquainted with plants and animals and their nutrition. A nutritional problem in plants often is passed on to the animal eating the plant, and eventually to the people eating the animals or plants or both[18]. Agricultural research background definitely is needed in a team effort to solve human nutritional diseases, a field that has been rather grossly neglected. It is difficult to experiment with humans but unlimited tests can be run with animals. Response of livestock, particularly the pig, to food and environmental changes is similar to that of humans. The pig is an expensive animal for experimentation so much of the work is done with rats.

Agricultural researchers in solving farm problems often make discoveries that also benefit people and the treatment of their diseases. Two of dozens of these examples are cited in the accompanying photographs, one of Dr. Karl Paul Link of the University of Wisconsin and the other of the late Dr. Selman A. Waksman of Rutgers University in New Jersey.

The colleges of veterinary science and medicine in the agricultural experiment stations have made immense contributions over the years to agriculture and the health and well being of the consumer.

Briefly, a sampling of these contributions are: Developed spinal anesthesia; devised the hypodermic needle injection technique; formulated immunizing techniques with toxoids for tetanus and diphtheria; developed catherizing in human surgery; solved botulism problems in the canning industry; found that human pellagra can be prevented by use of niacin; control of human hookworm with tetrachloroethylene; with reserpine studies developed tranquilizers for humans, plus numerous other contributions. *In summary,* over half of the U.S. veterinary profession, either

---

[18]Squibb, Robert V. (A tropical and temperate food nutritionist). Rutgers University, New Brunswick, N.J. Personal communication. 1977.

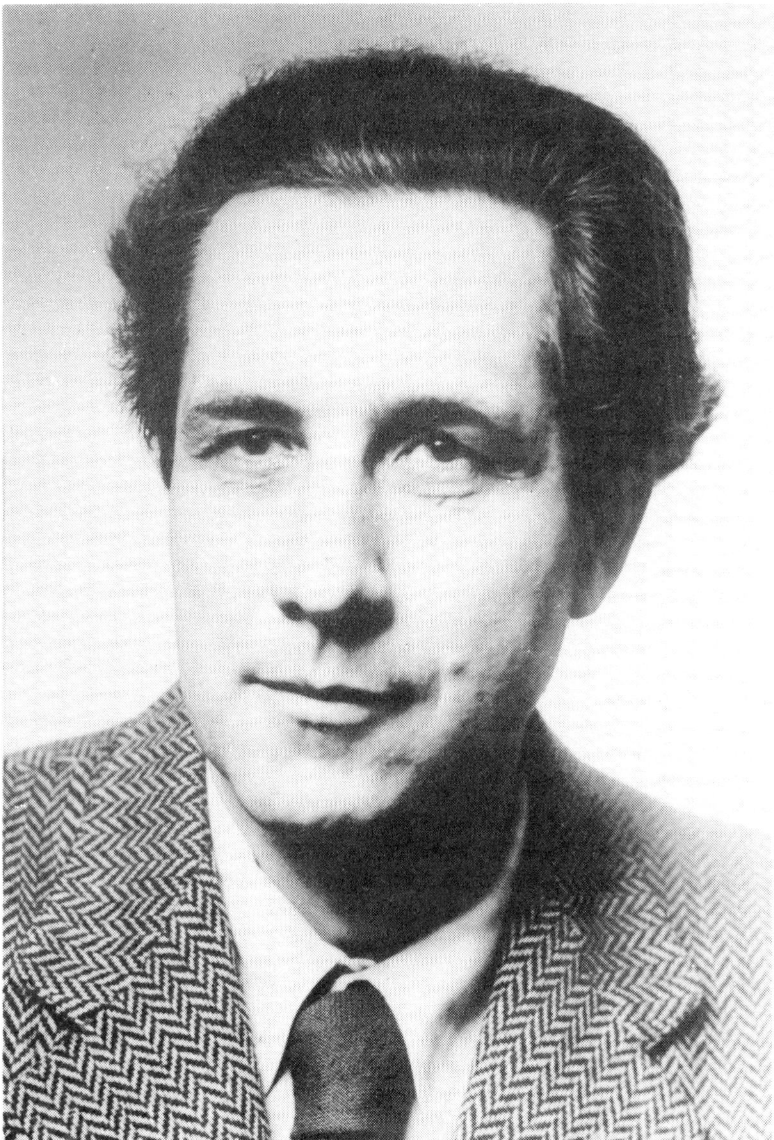

Dr. Karl Paul Link, a retired agricultural biochemist at the University of Wisconsin, Madison, discovered and helped develop the anticoagulant, *Dicoumarol,* now used to prevent blood clotting in humans. He first isolated 4-hydroxy-coumarin from spoiled sweet clover which was causing dairy cattle to bleed profusely when pricked by a barbed wire fence. This chemical also is used to control rats (Warfarin), who on ingesting it bleed to death internally. It also is used in South and Central America to control a predaceous vampire bat species on cattle.

directly or indirectly, contributes to human health and preventative medicine through their activities in livestock practice, regulatory disease control, and food inspection and research.

Funding New Research In Human Nutrition

There are many staff members in the agricultural experiment stations both domestic and foreign who are well qualified to help in solving human diseases, if so assigned. And you can be reasonably sure they would undertake the work with a missionary attitude. Actually, there are few diseases in agriculture at this time that are unsolved.

If agricultural staffs could be assigned along with medical researchers to work on human nutritional diseases, the botanist could advise on the classification and grouping of plants, the plant breeder can breed down or try to eliminate any toxic material in a plant, the chemist can remove the toxins from the processed product[19], the food scientist can modify the processing procedure, the plant pathologist and entomologist can evaluate and correct any disease or pest associated with the problem, the veterinarian and animal nutritionist can experiment with test animals, and the agronomist and horticulturist as well as the engineers can seek replacement crops and adjust or perfect the cultural and handling procedures, all to solve a human disease problem.

All we need is encouragement and *new funding* to do the job. We say "new funding" because the agricultural staffs already are fully occupied in the production of quality food. Private or industrial grants (in addition to state and Federal) for graduate student training are relatively economical and they serve two purposes: (a) accomplish needed research, and (b) help to train young people for the professional field of human nutrition. Private grants with "no strings attached" of $10,000 to $15,000 annually for two years (masters degree) or for three to four years (doctorate) can be negotiated easily with interested departments in agriculture or medicine. When "no strings" are attached (findings will not be patented), the university will not withdraw 35% or more of the grant for maintenance and administration. The grant will need to cover at least the salary and tuition of the graduate student. Any additional monies can be used for supplies and equipment. Trained PhD and MD staff also will be needed.

The "Nightshades Research Foundation" has been established with specific objectives listed on page 187. Trustees of the Foundation are convinced that several important human diseases are caused by improper diet and that the Nightshades are likely a key cause. If you wish to contribute to this worthy study, large or small, the trustees would be happy to hear from you.

We have enough leads in this book to keep dozens of researchers

[19]Laszlo, Somogy, PhD, Food Scientist, Sanford Res. Inst., Menlo Park; Ca., 94025, advises that solanine can be removed from a processed potato.

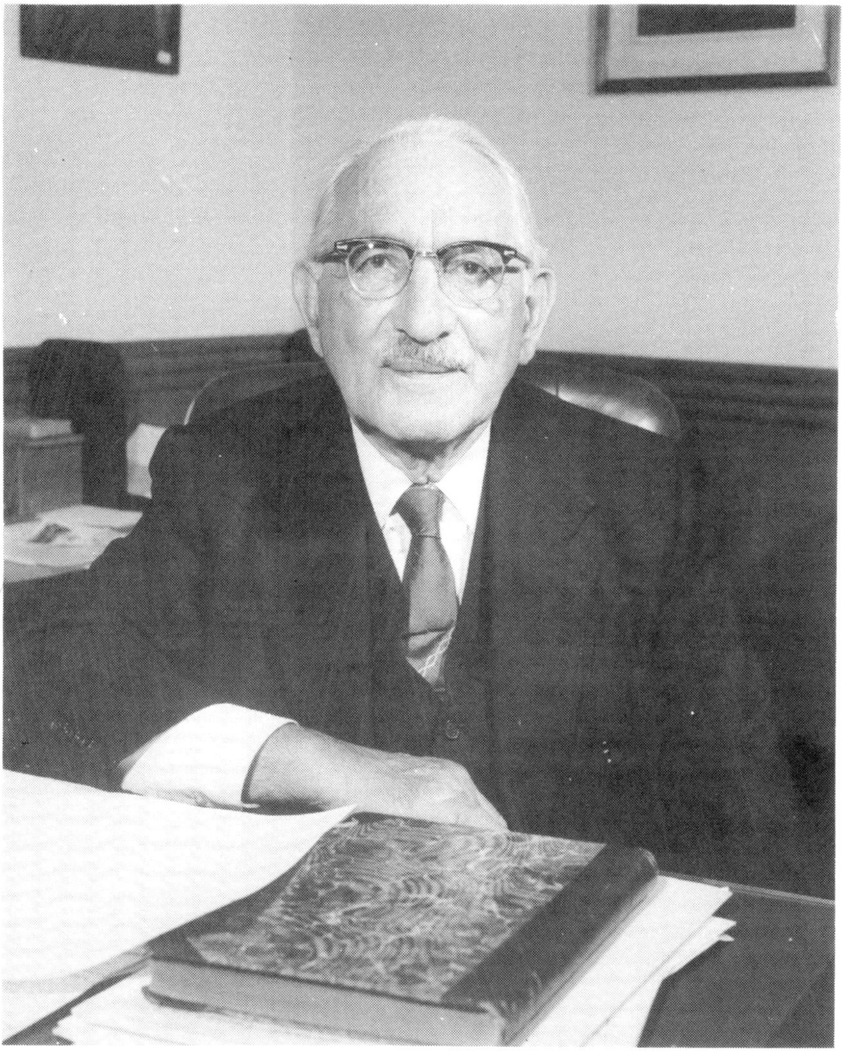

The late **Dr. Selman Abraham Waksman** (1888-1973), an agricultural soil biochemist at Rutgers University in New Jersey, isolated *streptomycin* from a soil fungus in 1943. Streptomycin became a major factor in almost eliminating tuberculosis of humans which had developed into serious proportions by the middle of this century. Dr. Waksman also developed *neomycin* used in treating many infectuous diseases of humans, animals and plants.

working productively for a long time. Did you ever check through The Merck Manual of human diseases[20], or any health manual, and note the numerous diseases for which there is no known cause and/or control? Many of the diseases are rather common and could be associated with the diet, a field as noted above that has been neglected. A low level subtle poisoning of the body, as with the *Solanaceae* toxins, could eventually result in a number of digestive, circulatory, nervous and structural diseases of humans, as with animals[21].

Since the first edition of this book in 1977, we are seeing an increasing number of items in the media urging more research in human nutrition to find the *causes* of cardiovascular and degenerative diseases, high blood pressure, heart attacks, and, above all, cancer. In 1978-79 the U. S. Department of Agriculture was asked to direct 15 million dollars toward research on human nutritional diseases, a first, since the Department has worked mainly on farm problems in the past.

In the 1980s over one billion dollars is being spent by the American Cancer Institute, mostly on treatment of cancer and little on finding the cause.

Impact

As indicated earlier, there may be a moderate impact of this Diet on the food and drug industries since only about 10% of the population suffers from arthritis. The impact of the tobacco-health situation has been only moderate on the usage of tobacco. Farmers in any event have been and are able and quick to switch to other annual crops if they are in demand and if they are bringing better net profits.

State and Federal agricultural experiment stations together with agricultural colleges, and their highly trained staffs, always have been ready and able to help farmers and industry make any needed shifts to other crops that can be grown in a given area. Also, these agencies are in a position to seek new crops[22] or by research make necessary adjustments in the current crops to keep the farmers, the markets and the consumers reasonably happy.

If there is a change in the production and movement of these crops, it likely will not be felt for 5 to 10 years.

---

[20]Holvey, Davis N. (Ed.) The Merck Manual of Diagnosis and Therapy. Merck Sharp and Dohme Research Laboratories, Rahway, N.J. 1964 pp. 1972.

[21]Kingsbury, John M. Poisonous plants of the United States and Canada. Prentice-Hall Inc., Englewood Cliffs, N.J. 275-294. 1964.

[22]The Division of Plant Introduction, U.S. Dept. of Agriculture, Glendale, Maryland, has a staff of explorers circulating over the world in search of new crops that may have an economical use in the United States.

CHAPTER II

The Childers' Diet

The Diet is simple, but not easy for most people. It is a control — not a cure! The Diet is not a cure in the sense that you can go back to eating and using the nightshades again!

For your test period, *you must completely avoid the nightshades listed below for at least 3 months* — better 6 to 12 months. *Complete abstinence — NO half-hearted approach!* Otherwise, little or no results. After the test period, you may wish to go off the Diet for a week to 10 days to see if your problems return or worsen.

Please avoid:

WHITE POTATO

TOMATO

EGGPLANT

PEPPERS, ALL KINDS (Including pimiento, Cayenne, paprika, chili) Black and white pepper are okay*

ALL BY-PRODUCTS OF ABOVE CROPS

TOBACCO**

Precaution: Read "INGREDIENTS" on all cans, bottles, boxes and packages to avoid foods on grocery counters with tomato sauce and paste, paprika, red and green peppers, eggplant, white potato and white potato starch or flour. Be suspicious of "spices" and "spiced" salt, "Natural Flavoring." They may contain paprika.

---

*Black and white pepper, *Piper nigrum, L.,* belong to a different family of plants, *Piperaceae,* and can be used in the diet. Dried berries of black pepper are the peppercorns of trade and white pepper is the dried ground seeds divested of their coats. The red pepper (pimiento, paprika, chili, cayenne, are essentially ground red peppers after seed removal) and green (sweet) peppers, *Capsicum* spp., belong to the *Solanaceae* family of plants, the nightshades, and *are to be avoided.*

**Cooperating smokers have not been able to free themselves completely of aches and pains so long as they are smoking. But they have reduced them appreciably by avoiding the other nightshades. Smokers should try to stop smoking completely, "cold turkey."

Foods Containing Nightshades

Table 1 lists most of the foods on grocery shelves that may contain the nightshades. After a few weeks or months, it should become second nature for you to be aware of where the nightshades are likely to occur and to avoid them automatically. Always read the "Ingredients" on containers.

Table 1. Foods in which nightshades may be found on grocery shelves. Always check "Ingredients" on containers.

DON'T EAT POTATO IN*

Baby foods, some, canned	Pierogies
Beef stew, hash	Pies, beef, chicken, turkey, frozen
Biscuits, some (potato flour)	Pancakes, some
Breads, some	Potato "Nuts" (skins, deep fried)
Candies, some	Sauce, Taco
Cakes, some	Passover foods, some
Casseroles	Pork sausage
Chips, potato, snack (Prothin's)	Soups, many, dry, canned pea-green, split, beef
Chowder, clam	Starch, some
Consomme	Stuffings
Dog food meats, some canned**	Stews
Doughnuts, some	Tuna, broth
Dumplings	Vegetables, mixed, canned, frozen
Fish cakes, some	"Vegetable Starch"
Gravies (thick)	Wafers, some
Flour, some	
Meat balls, loaf, stews	

DON'T EAT TOMATO IN

Baby foods, meats, others, canned	Italian, most frozen, canned, dry foods
Barbecue sauces	Delicatessen foods, many
Beans, baked, canned	Macaroni shells, canned
Beef, Tacos, stews, canned, pies, soups	Meat loaf
Chips, Tortilla	Rice, Spanish, canned
Cabbage, frozen, stuffed	Salad dressings, most
Chow mein, canned	Salisbury steaks, frozen
Chicken mixes prepared for fried chicken	Sauces, Ronzoni, taco, cocktail, steak, many others
Dinners, TV, weight watchers, Oriental, frozen, most	Soups, tomato, chicken gumbo, beef, vegetable, dry, etc.
Fillets, herring, some	Spaghetti & meat balls, canned
Gravies	Tuna, broth
Hamburger Helper	Vegetable juice, canned, mixed

*Glut of potatoes on the market may result in more potatoes shunted to flour and processing.
**This may account for arthritis in pets; they also get nightshades in table scraps.

DON'T EAT PEPPERS — RED, GREEN, PAPRIKA[1], ETC. IN (Black or White Pepper okay)

Artichoke hearts, canned
Baby foods, some meats
Bologna
Bread crumbs, some Italian
Bow ties and Kaska
Cauliflower, pickled, spiced
Cheese, some
Chicken, a la King, frozen, canned; hot pickup; pies, chow mein, canned
Chips, corn, Tortilla
Cookies, seasoned
Coffee cake, some
Crabs, frozen, deviled, miniature
Chinese mixed vegetables
Delicatessen preparations, many (note red sprinkled paprika)
Dinners, frozen, Oriental, many
Dips, snack, enchilada, bean, sandwich, many
Egg noodles, Chinese
Eggplant appetizer
Fish, precooked, frozen; cakes, frozen
Fillets, herring, smoked; and shrimp frozen, breaded
Gefilte fish
Gravies, several
Ham glaze, baked
Herb Teas (Capsicum)
Hot dogs, weiners
Hot mix, pickled
Herring, smoked, pickled
Italian foods, most
Matzah Balls
Meat loaf; luncheon, smoked; many cold; tenderizers
Mayonnaises, most
Olives, stuffed, salad
Onion rings, frozen, soups
Passover foods
Peanuts, bottled, roasted, some butter
Peppers, frozen, stuffed, crushed red dry, Rice and Bell, pickled chili, cayenne, pimientos
Pies, chicken, meat, turkey, frozen, many
Relishes
Rice, Chinese, fried, seasoned, Spanish w/sweet pepper bits
Raisin bread, some
Rarebit, Welsh
Roquefort cheese, if mayonnaise used
Sauces, Barbecue, meat frozen breakfast meat, some frozen vegetable and Chinese, Sloppy Joe
Salts, some seasoned
Salad dressings, many
Sausages, frozen, others
Sardines, Spanish, International**
Seasoning mixes
Shake and Bake mixes
Shrimp croquettes, scampi, frozen
Snacks, crackers, many
Some sodas and cokes
Soups, many
Spreads, sandwich, cracker
Tacos, beef
Tobasco
Tuna, in broth
Veal patties, frozen
Vegetables, International frozen, juices, mixes**
Vitamin pills, some "C", multiple

---

[1]Be aware that linaments and ointments may have hot pepper in them and it can be absorbed through the skin and taken into the blood system. Some cough lozenges may contain hot pepper. Pills, drops, may contain nightshades, as Lomotil, Belladonna, Atropine, Scopalamine (sleeping pills). Be suspicious of "Natural Flavoring."

**Foreign canned foods coming into USA may not list all ingredients, if any.

THE DIET

Some Substitutes For Nightshades

There are dozens of foods to eat other than the nightshades. People often say, "What else is there to eat?" After a period of time on the diet you begin to "forget" the nightshades, more or less "lose" appetite for them. The following are suggested substitutions. You will discover others.

WHITE POTATO SUBSTITUTES

Sweet potato
Rice
Jerusalem artichoke*
Noodles
Carrots**
Grits
Corn
Squash
Pumpkin
Rice (French) Frys

Rutabaga
Turnips
Parsnips
Radishes
Onions,
  creamed,
  rings
Beans
Shallots
Dasheen

Yautia
Manioc
Plantain (chips too)
Kohlrabi
Bread, other flour
  products
Chick peas,
  mashed with butter
Others
Yams***

PEPPERS, TOMATO, EGGPLANT SUBSTITUTES

Fruits
Cucumber
Cauliflower
Cabbage
Lettuce
Brussel sprouts
Radishes
Celery
Black Pepper
White Pepper

Endive
Melons****
Cress
Parsley
Chives
Collards
Watermelon****
Okra
Artichoke (Globe)
Chinese cabbage

Dandelion
Garlic
Onion, bunch
Olives
  (No pimientos)
Leek
Squash
Chicory
Other leafy vegetables
Others

---

*Jerusalem artichokes are sunflower-like, easy to grow, and produce tubers abundantly.

**Carrots have some ardent health-food followers; they drink quantities of the juice daily, eat raw carrots, etc. Research indicates that carrots may help to counteract solanine in the nightshades.

***Some tropical yams are toxic to humans; avoid those with acrid flavor.

****Excess melons in season may "bother" some people.

Vitamins

If you are eating regularly and normally, there is a good chance that vitamin pills and supplements are not needed. Much of the "need" for pills is created through pressure advertising.

There is a danger of overdosing with A and D vitamin pills and vitamin additives (U.S. News and World Report, July 15, 1974, p. 63). Excess vitamin "A" can cause enlarged liver and spleen, low-key pain in liver region, and falling hair. Pfeiffer notes that excess vitamin A also can cause bursitis, red discoloration of gums, itchy skin, muscle stiffness, and intracranial pressure (bad headaches). Excess vitamin D may cause calcium deposits in the main arteries, in joints, and in the kidneys resulting in renal failure and elevated blood pressure which sometimes is fatal.* Cooperators have noted excess E may cause urinary problems.

Vitamin C pills, surprising to say, were found by several cooperators to cause sore feet and tendons, swollen toes, inflamed joints, sore jaws and other problems. When the pills were stopped, the problems went away; when started again, they returned. Some brands of vitamin C pills contain paprika as a "natural" source of C. Ascorbic acid (vitamin C) is derived from potato or corn starch in some brands, but it is not certain if those made from potato starch can carry the nightshade effect over into the ascorbic acid pills. Some cooperators complained of large red and purple spots forming on their limbs when high dosages of vitamin C were taken voluntarily or recommended. Other cooperators did not complain about vitamin C pills taken at a daily minimum or irregularly, or at what could be considered an excess for other cooperators. Cod liver oil which has A and D was found to cause fuzziness and feeling "rotten" by some people. There obviously is a difference among people in their reactions to vitamin pills and supplements and this would need to be considered in assessing what has been said above.

On the other hand, we have some cooperators who apparently have responded to multimineral, multivitamin, calcium, alfalfa, hormone and other pills when nothing else seemed to help their ailments. For example, one cooperator felt tired, had leg aches, and a goiter swelling that was corrected by taking multimineral pills *only as needed* and not day in and day out. If a pill seems to give a response at first, it is unwise to take an abundance of them daily or even the minimum daily since there is a good chance of creating another problem.

It may take 3 to 6 months to recover from an overdose of vitamins. Vitamin pills and supplements tend to be oversold in advertising. It is best to spend your money on good and varied food rather than on pills and supplements. As you gain time with the Diet, you should be able to gradually reduce as many of the pills as you can; then omit all of them if at

*Be aware of possible sensitivity to and body accumulation of Vitamin D from fortified milk, cheese, etc., and from multiple vitamin pills and sunning. See Chap. VI by Dr. George Davis.

all possible. The body was not made for the many pills some people are taking today. Also, some people take large doses of vitamins so they can eat and drink carelessly! Not Good!

Read labels carefully and watch buildup of added vitamins A, D and C in prepared foods and drinks.

Exercise

Exercise of any kind helps blood circulation, tissue repair, and the carrying away of toxins through the kidneys. Massaging of the tender bone and muscle areas improves blood circulation, as do sunning, hot baths and heat pads. Golf, walking, tennis, jogging, or "running around" on the job all stimulate blood circulation and help to get quicker relief while on the Diet.

The Potato

The white potato needs special comment. The potato is often the last nightshade to be given up by Dieters. It is the most common food, cooked in many ways, on the breakfast, lunch and dinner dishes. It is difficult to resist. Most people cannot believe that such a white, clean, innocent looking, good tasting and easy-to-digest food can cause aches and pains. The potato has a delayed action, giving first a tranquilizing effect, then an ache or pain setting in within a few hours or a day to two later. Severity of pain varies with the amount eaten. But for sensitive people, just bits of potato, cooked, or mixed in other foods as flour or paste, is enough to keep the problem active.

Other Possible Food Offenders

The nightshades are by far the key offenders, and based on animal research, could be responsible for subtle bone, tendon, tooth, and tissue deterioration with time. Some cooperators have complained of aches and pains after eating asparagus, beets, spinach, rhubarb (will clean pans), sweet cherries, *chocolate* and some wines and liquors, particularly when used daily or in excess. People will vary in susceptibility. Some cooperators consider peas an offender, but this could be due to green berries of a nightshade weed being harvested in the commercial field with the peas. Employees remove most of these berries on the sorting belt or by use of a selective herbicide in the field. Melons in excess may create a problem.

There may be other offenders and we would be glad to hear from you. Coffee and chocolate may cause skin eruptions and headless pimples mostly on the face with some people. Artificial coffee cream and instant coffee may cause digestive problems. Some cooperators complain of corn products and wheat flour (could it be potato flour?). Go easy with milk (can cause colitis) and milk products, particularly cheese (contains vitamin D, possibly paprika). Sodas labeled "Natural Flavoring" may contain paprika. Excess pork, eggs, sweets and citrus (combined with vitamin C in pills) have caused complaints.

Restaurants, Banquets, Hospitals, Airlines, Picnics

Study the menu. Instead of white potato, ask for rice, two vegetables, a salad, or a sweet potato if listed. Many people are weight reducing and the waitress understands, "no potato". Ask for grits if available.

Ask for a tossed salad *without* tomatoes or peppers, or ask for hearts-of-lettuce. Most salad dressings have tomato or hot pepper in them in one form or another. Roquefort or oil-and-vinegar are O.K., provided a "cheap" brand of Roquefort has not been made with mayonnaise (containing paprika). French, Russian, Thousand Island and Italian dressings have tomato and maybe hot pepper in them.

Pretty red *paprika* often is sprinkled over fish dishes and seafoods generally. You also may find it on macaroni salads and many of the delicatessen foods. Watch for olives with pimiento peppers in them.

Avoid meat sauces, most of which have tomato, maybe hot pepper in them. Use black pepper and salt instead. A fruit cup is safer than a soup.

Watch for tomato cooked into green beans, limas, zucchini, cucumbers, hamburger, meat loaf, other foods. You may be able to smell or taste the tomato if you cannot see it, and immediately avoid these dishes. Eat more, or take more from the buffet counter of other foods, maybe even bread or desserts.

You will find it pays to be finicky.

Banquets can be a real problem where you are served the same meal across-the-board. Lay aside the tomato or pepper. If the potato is baked, as often is the case, open it, spread it, and smear it as if you "did" eat some. Friends may think you are dieting, and you are! Watch for paprika and nightshades cooked and mixed with other foods. Sometimes, with a hidden nightshade, you cannot help yourself and must endure the aches and pains.

In hospitals you usually have a choice on the menu before food is served. Avoid the nightshades and order more of others. It is highly important to avoid the nightshades when trying to get well. Here is a place vitamin pills, one a day, C or multiple, may be in order. Vitamin C is a healing vitamin.

In nursing homes it is difficult to get the food you want, but a sympathetic nutritionist often will work with you and the chef to serve you foods without nightshades.

On airlines you do not have much choice. Do the best you can, do without, or bring a bag! Watch paprika on peanuts, in spicy sausage, potato water in gravies.

At picnics, nightshades tend to be "everywhere" — tomatoes and peppers in the vegetable salad, potato or macaroni salad sprinkled with pretty red paprika, brown beans with tomato sauce, potato chips and snacks with paprika on or in them, red pimiento peppers in olives, barbeque sauce on the meats, etc. All that may be left for you are breads, cakes, desserts and maybe a drink. Pick up what you can or try to brush aside as much tomato sauce as you can (this could be too much for some people), and delay for a "hamburger" afterward! Or, pay the price in pain.

Eating at a Friend's House

Warn the hostess beforehand that you are unable to eat white potato, tomato, eggplant, or peppers in any form. "Allergies!" This is better than "picking" at your food later with embarrassment. With some families they can hardly cook a meal without using the nightshades in one form or another. And this creates a real problem that must be faced — or be ready to endure the aches and pains later.

Double Checking

After you have been on the Diet for 3 to 6 months, you may wish to go back to eating the nightshades for a week or two to see if the aches, pains and other problems return. You may "slip" unavoidably. In either case, it may help to convince you that you are on the right track. But it usually takes another two or three weeks to eliminate the problem again, depending upon how much and how long you partook of the nightshades.

Duration of Test Period

It usually takes at least 3 months to get the toxins out of your system and for the body to start recovering. You may see benefits within 4 to 6 weeks. The aches and pains disappear *very slowly,* and suddenly you realize they are gone. Where there has been a sprain, a bruise, a bone break, surgery, or tissue damage, it may take several months or more for the tenderness to disappear from these areas. If the damage is of long-standing, and joints or vertebrae have fused, or fingers and toes gnarled, the nerves may be pressed and pains may continue until surgery is performed. Arthritic problems seem to settle first in damaged areas of the body. This is probably due to a sprain or surgery cutting or pulling apart of the blood vessels and nerves. Hence, the toxins settle in these "dead ends" and it takes awhile for them to move out. When aches and pains of arthritis are worse during cool wet weather, this could be due to poorer blood circulation and a slower movement of nightshade toxins through the kidneys into the urine. Most of the cooperators on this Diet, when rigid, find after a few weeks or months that change of weather makes little or no difference.

Remember again that this Diet is a control. If you go back to the nightshades, your troubles are "refunded!"

After a year or two on the Diet, avoiding the nightshades becomes a part of the daily routine without much thought since it becomes second nature to know where the nightshades are likely to occur. Also, the body seems to settle down from "ups and downs" that may occur with most people for the first 6 to 12 months on the Diet, perhaps due to getting bits of hidden nightshades by mistake, and also the body may need this time to adjust.

Salt

Do we have adequate research backing on the use of salt in the human diet? Is a completely salt-free diet healthful? Can a "salt" problem in health be due to another factor, or a combination of factors? Any toxin, such as those in nightshades, can cause edema (water accumulation in tissues, etc.). The nightshade effects on edema in some people could be a reason for suggesting salt-free diets.

The farmer and agricultural researcher look at the need for salt, essentially table salt (sodium chloride), somewhat differently than the medical doctor. Dairymen place a block of sodium chloride among their cattle to provide the animals with sodium, needed in high milk production. In fact, the animal appetite demands it. Wild animals also can be seen seeking salt where it is available. People perspiring on hot days, as on the farm or in construction, eat salt pills regularly to keep from becoming exhausted and weak.

If you suddenly become weak from heavy perspiration while mowing the lawn, e.g., place a teaspoon of table salt in a glass of warm water and drink it; within minutes your strength returns to normal.

With a tight head cold, you can often open the nose by sucking a medium strength table salt solution (gargling w/strong sol.) from the palm of your hand up through the nasal channels into the throat, clear the nose, do it again; once/2-3 hours. Our blood, perspiration, tears, and urine are salty. In Central Africa away from the sea, people have become so in need of salt that they drank cattle urine. Bloch[2] attributes the low population density in Central Africa to the environmental inadequacy of sodium chloride. Charles E. Weber[3] has associated inadequate potassium salts with some of the aches and pains of arthritis. A balance is needed in the body among the salts — sodium, potassium, magnesium, others. When one element is out of balance, troubles arise.

Note: Our body contains a half pound of salt, enough to fill several shakers.

Has a fad of salt-free diets developed over the years without adequate research backing? There appears to be a need for more study in this area[4].

---

[2]Bloch, M. R. The social influence of salt. Journ. Amer. Dietetic Ass'n 25 (4). p. 304, 1964.
[3]Weber, Chas. E. Arthritis as a chronic potassium deficiency. 22 pp. Industrial Research Co., Mt. Horeb Rd. Plainfield, N. J. 1965. See also, "K etiology for mesenchyme degeneration. Journ. Theor. Biol. 29:327-8. 1970, and J. Appl. Nutr. Spring Ed. 26: No. 12, p. 41. 1974.
[4]See Young, G. The Essence of Life — Salt. National Geographic. 380-401. Sept. 1977.

Red Meat and Eggs

Red meat is the best source of endurance energy. It more nearly resembles the tissues of your body. Fish and fowl are deficient in a few of the amino acids found in your body. Football coaches always request big steaks for their teams before a game. They would not recommend a meal of, e.g., tuna fish, cottage cheese, tossed salad, mushrooms and an apple, even though each has a definite place in the diet.

There is nothing wrong with one or two eggs a day, if no allergies are involved[1]. Most of the food requirements of life are in eggs and the cholesterol can be countered by daily consumption of fresh fruits and vegetables that contain a key item, pectin[2]. Some fat in meats is not harmful and is a good source of energy, but a substantial diet of fatty meats and foods is questionable. Most of the fat around steaks can be cut away and left on the plate.

The senior author has spent a sabbatical leave visiting dozens of countries around the world, studying agriculture in general and fruit growing in particular. The healthiest, most progressive and largest people are living in areas where the land is fertile and good water is plentiful. In other words, the people are where the food is and where agriculture, the biggest industry in the world, is active and thriving. The United States of America has by far the best food and particularly red meat (steaks). This, of course, is due to good natural resources, but mainly to the efficient farmers trained by the agricultural colleges and extension services and backed by the excellent research of the agricultural experiment stations over the country. The free enterprise system has been a factor encouraging competition among farmers to produce the most and the best.

Pills, Drugs, Alcohol

To relieve pain, the use of pills, alcohol and perhaps hard drugs are an easy "out". Unfortunately, pills and exercise seem to be the only approach left for most doctors, or massaging and bone treatment by others. Surgery, can be effective in advanced cases. Acupuncture has been temporarily effective for some people, but rarely permanently, according to replies from many cooperators. Gold shots and copper bracelets are questionable. Cortisone has been temporarily effective but has bad side effects when continued. Some cooperators on the diet who have taken cortisone have worsened. Why, we do not know. DMSO (dimethyl sulfoxide) and cocaine (Esterene) are short-term pain killers with eventual problems. Pills, drugs and alcohol only soothe you while the disease worsens.

---

[1]Eggs on successive days have caused two cooperators sore jaws, swollen necks.

[2]Fisher, Hans, P. Grimminger, E. R. Sostman and M. K. Brush. Dietary pectin and blood cholesterol. The Journal of Nutrition. *86:*(1) 113. 1965.

By avoiding the nightshades and their by-products, you should be able to reduce gradually the intake of pills. Most of these pills slow you down, cause ups and downs, make you sleepy, blur mentality, tire you, can have severe side effects, and if taken in excess may induce sleeplessness. It is best to reduce, then stop them completely as pains subside. You may have forgotten how it is to feel really good, be ambitious and enjoy life.

Some pain killers are highly addictive to some people, as alcohol, cocaine and valium. In extreme cases of addiction, it is wise to go to a clinic to stop them and get a new start. If you become an alcoholic or drug addict, long years of experience have shown that attending and taking part in AA (Alcoholics Anonymous) meetings is the only effective control. Alcoholism is a recognized disease. Excess drinking may result in alcoholic neuritis — aches and pains in muscles and joints that may be diagnosed as a form of arthritis. The AA technique of not picking up a drink a day at a time and going to AA and Smoke-End meetings regularly, may also work for addiction to drugs and tobacco.

Fasting

Fasting is an approach some doctors use to pinpoint foods that may be causing allergies, or arthritis symptoms. The patient fasts for four or five days, then starts eating foods, beginning e.g. with meat and adding others one by one until a "kickback" is noted. Some foods as a potato, however, have a delayed action and aches may not appear for 1-3 days after eaten. This must be taken into consideration.

One New Brunswick, N.J. cooperator tells about a friend who got lost at sea and ate only fish that he could catch for several days. His arthritic symptoms disappeared during this episode, but returned after he began to eat "shore" food.

Rheumatologists at Linkoping Regional Hospital in Sweden have reported that fasting can afford temporary relief from rheumatoid arthritis. Fifteen rheumatoid patients fasted for 7-10 days while 10 other rheumatoid patients served as controls. All patients were observed over 9 weeks. While fasting, the study subjects experienced a significant reduction in pain, joint swelling and joint stiffness compared with the control subjects. But a few days after stopping the fast the disease symptoms returned for the study subjects. Results were published in a 1979 issue of Lakartidningen.

Working Wives, Mothers

Working women may have a difficult time with this Diet. Meals need to be planned or prepared ahead. Today, rather typically, she may call her husband or son at 4:00 p.m., "Pick up four hamburgers, big ones, a big bag of French fries, two milk shakes, five pies and a big cup of cole slaw (with green peppers chopped in) at the burger restaurant, and also get a couple of bottles of ketchup". Or mother calls daughter just home from school, "Put four potatoes in the oven to bake, take a steak out of the freezer to thaw and prepare a salad. There are plenty of tomatoes, peppers, radishes and some celery and carrots in the refrigerator. See if we have enough French dressing, or Russian. Call me back to get anything you need. I'll be home about 5:15."

It also is quick and easy to put prepared foods on the table from the supermarket and many of them contain nightshades in one form or another. Hence, working women using this Diet may have to do more home cooking with considerable advance planning to make the Diet work!

Husbands!

Women seem generally to take more interest in what they eat. Their health and figure seem to be more important than with men. Men will eat almost anything put before them (a bit of an exaggeration), and can be a problem in trying to get them to adhere to a diet. As indicated before, if they hurt badly enough, they pay attention. Sometimes wives must take all the nightshades in any form out of the house (but men will pick them up at lunch or banquets or in travelling). Some wives put their husbands on the Diet without their knowing it, then explain what happened later. Maybe this is the reason there are so many widows around today! For many men, some women, a Diet is just too much bother. It is easier to take pills when the pain gets bad enough!

Nurses

There are dozens of nurses on this Diet — and happy to find something other than pills for their crippling and pains. We have heard from a few nurses who have recovered from arthritic problems but under no condition are they able to convince their doctors to even try the Diet. Most nurses will pass the information on to clients. Here again, a difference between women and men.

Sports and Nightshades

The nightshades with some people, and perhaps with most people without their knowing it, tend to stiffen and slow muscle movement, their actions and reactions. When used in "excess," the nightshades may cause muscle spasms as a "charley horse" in the thigh, a "crick" in the back, "trick joints", or even an heart arrest. The glycoalkaloids in the nightshades are known to cause paralysis to a degree. Bone breaks and sprains on the football field, e.g., could be due in some cases to a muscle spasm and a failure of the muscles under strain to protect the bone. It is well known that shortage of breath and quicker fatigue are associated with the use of tobacco. For any temporary stimulation from nicotine, there is a "let-down" later. Hence, most coaches discourage their teams from using tobacco. Back in the early 1900s, the author can remember his father who was center on the Missouri University football team, telling him on two occasions that his coach would not let the team use hot pepper during training, apparently because of the same problem with tobacco. Heavy tomato consumption has developed only in recent years in the USA, but potatoes back in the early 1900s were largely mashed or fried in skillets and not eaten baked, as today, with the peel which is high in solanine.

Knee, arm and leg injuries are common in the heavy sports as football and hockey. Arthritis frequently develops after injury, eventually disabling the player for future participation in sports. We have seen middle-aged cooperators on the Diet recover to youth and agility of a 20-yr old; there really is no good reason for athletes to retire from the game at 40 yrs. The No-Nightshades Diet should help these athletes to recover from injuries and stay agile for another decade or two after 40 yrs of age.

It could be of interest to athletes to try not eating the nightshades before and during sports events to see if their performance is better and more consistent. Coaches also may be interested in trying the No-Nightshades meals during the sports season. Hundreds of cooperators have indicated to us that while on the Diet, they have noted markedly increased strength, endurance and mental alertness. The nightshade foods actually are mild drug or narcotic crops, as is tobacco.

Libido

Several cooperators have indicated improved libido on the Diet. This could be due to a generally improved health condition when free from the nightshade toxins. In a press release spring 1980, Drs. George Ehrlich of Temple Univeristy and Jesse E. Potter, Chicago, noted that in their experience with 220 patients at the Moss Rehabilitation Hospital,

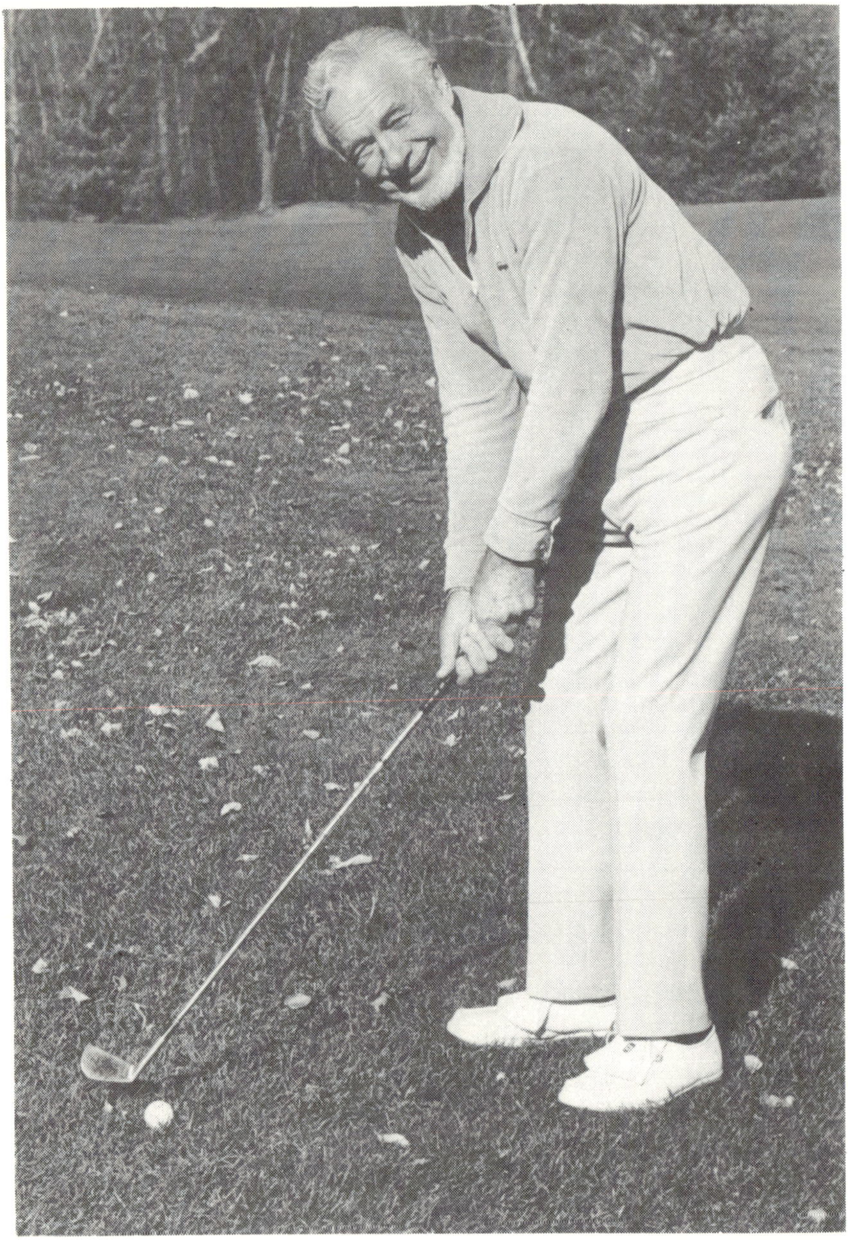

Prof. Raymond P. Korbobo, Landscape Design Specialist, WCBS-TV, Rutgers University, New Brunswick, N. J. was having aches, pains and stiffness in his legs, back, shoulders, arms and hands. He could not grasp the golf club solidly. He liked all nightshades, mainly white potatoes with skins (high in solanine).

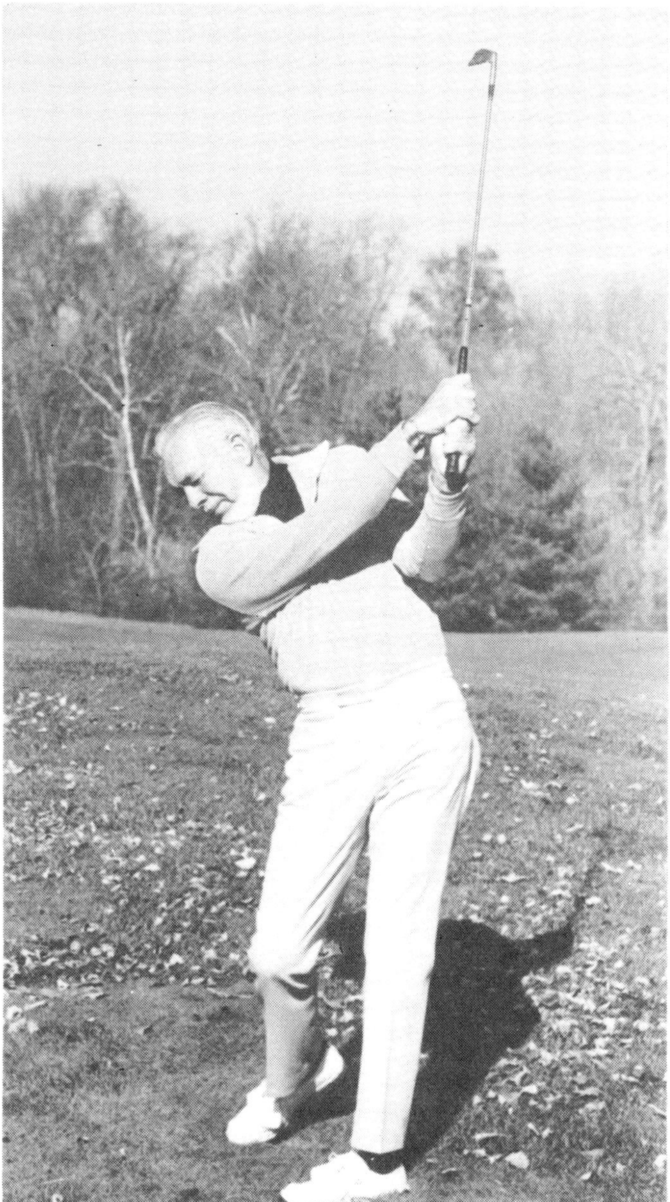

On the Diet, Prof. Korbobo can move nimbly and has a lower golf score. Diet cooperators in their teens and twenties also report better performance in sports and recreational activities. (New Brunswick Home News.)

Philadelphia, there was a 70% positive response to "intense sexual stimulation which provided 4 to 6 hrs of pain relief from joint disease". Sexual activity probably stimulates the adrenal glands to produce more cortisone, the hormone used to treat arthritics. A healthy sex life undoubtedly is significant in any program for better health.

Running Down a Food Problem

People vary in undesirable responses to food, other things. If you have a skin problem, a headache, or aches and pains that come and go, or is bad then not-so-bad, keep track of what you put into your mouth or are doing. When it is bad, trace back. By the process of elimination, sooner or later you may be able to pinpoint the culprit. This is the way we discovered the relation between aches and pains and the nightshades. It may take a few weeks, a few months, or a year, but it could be worth the effort. The culprit frequently is something you like very much and are eating or using in excess. The body tends to develop rejection symptoms under these conditions.

Be aware that a nightshade, particularly paprika, is likely to creep into your food at any time and you may ascribe a problem to another food or drink when it is the delayed action of the nightshade. With potato, e.g., there is a mild tranquilizing effect after eating it, but the ache or pain may not appear til a day or two later. A sizable "bite" of hot pepper, however, may be apparent within minutes, first in a tingling sensation in the chest or itching or irritation, then later an ache or pain setting in.

Some people think after being on the Diet for awhile, they can eat a potato or tomato and not be bothered, but these people usually continue taking an assortment of pills to correct discomfort or low-key aches.

People are all different genetically, the same as their fingerprints. You may be able to solve your own problem quickly and inexpensively by carefully studying your responses to food, drink and the environment around you. Where there is a pain, the body is "trying to tell you something is wrong". It is best to find the *cause* and correct it as soon as possible, rather than to kill the pain with pills while the problem worsens.

Practice Moderation, Variation

It is wise to eat and drink in moderation. Excesses may lead to allergies, as the body tends to develop rejection symptoms. Variation of meal makeup from day to day not only makes them more interesting and tasty, but also may avoid buildup of a problem with a food such as beets, spinach and asparagus, where cooperators have developed a "kickback" on eating them three or four days straight — in season. Excess sugar results in tooth cavities, blurred sight, fuzziness, and loss of vigor and endurance.

Junk Foods

For children in school, obviously too much sugar is not good or substituting a candy bar for a meal. Fruit machines would be better than most of the dispensing machines found in public places.

In the local area of New Jersey we often receive phone calls about a child suffering from some form of arthritis. In checking on food intake we usually find that they spend a lot of time at the fast food places where French fries, hamburgers and hot dogs with tomato sauce, tomatoes and hot pepper predominate. They may "live" on pizza pies. If we are able to get the child to avoid the nightshades completely, he soon recovers.

Acid Stomach

Some people seem to have more of a problem with an acid stomach developing after meals than others. A neutralizer such as Tums carried in the company's small plastic box is one solution. You will need to pick the brand that works best for you.

Acid stomach is aggravated by over-eating, eating between meals, by certain foods as hot pepper and tomatoes, going to bed "on a full stomach", some drinks as alcohol and coffee between meals and before food of last meal is digested. Most people are able eventually to pinpoint foods and drinks that affect them personally. Then there are people who seem never to complain of an acid stomach.

Diarrhea, Constipation

An effective method of stopping diarrhea is to reduce the liquid intake to almost nothing, taking a sip of water only when the urge is strong. A day or two of reduced water intake often will solve the problem. When the system is constantly flushed with liquid, the medication or the natural countering by the body does not have a chance to work. Banana is a recommended fruit in the tropics.

For constipation a ripe apple or any fresh fruit, eaten before or after a meal is effective in keeping the system open. Regular use of over-advertized medication to keep the system open may create the problem. For most people bowels will move when ready. Worrying only aggravates it. Forget it!

An Occasional Problem

Occasionally, we have a cooperator who is trying numerous things to regain good health or get rid of aches and pains, other problems. He may be taking as many as 100 pills a day (the extreme) and switching from one "health food" to another. Then he goes on this diet, but gets little if any results or they come very slowly. This could be due to an "over shadowing" effect of these other measures, or there could be another health problem dominating.

Some specialists may tend to go overboard on pain killers and other medicines to the point of actually causing the patient discomfort over and above the arthritic problem. Overdosing with vitamin pills and supplements is a common problem. The chiropractors and osteopaths sometimes are more successful in helping arthritics since they do not believe in drugs. There are some 150 of the latter doctors using the Diet with their standard treatments with favorable results. Several MDs are using the Diet on themselves to get relief and to help them continue in their profession and quite a number are testing the Diet on their patients.

It appears that the nightshades could be the "shadow" the medical profession has been "fighting" for years without knowing the basic culprit. Arthritis seems to be a warning symptom of other diseases subtly developing in the body, as hardening of the arteries, breakdown of organs, mental and cardiac problems and possibly cancer, in which all nightshades, including tobacco, may be playing a part.

Today, there is too much confusion in the media — newspapers, magazines, TV, radio — on just what you should do to solve health problems. We are extremely short on good basic well-conducted unbiased research on key problems of health, particularly in the field of human nutrition.

A Nutritional Diet Without Nightshades

Many people are "lost" at first as to what foods to buy and eat when they must omit the nightshades from their meals. After a little study, however, they find the problem is not much of a problem. There are dozens of other fruits and vegetables just as good or better.

Robert Bingham, MD Nutritionist of Yorba Linda, California 92686, has prepared a Nightshade-Free diet for some 300 of his patients at the Esperanza Intercommunity Hospital, and has given us permission to repeat it here. He says that all 300 of the patients on which the nightshades-free Diet has been tested have improved. But he also is using a number of other treatments as a part of his program for arthritics. In Table 2 breakfasts are indicated in the top tier of meals by week days, lunch in the middle tier and dinners at the base with respective desserts.

Table 2. Dr. Bingham's ESPERANZA INTERCOMMUNITY HOSPITAL

SUNDAY	MONDAY	TUESDAY
grape juice oats fr. toast w/ honey butter milk, 8 oz. hot beverage	orange juice granola hardbld. eggs rye toast w/ butr/diet jel. milk, 8 oz. hot beverage	cranby. juice malt-o-meal poached egg ww toast, butter diet jelly milk, 8 oz. hot beverage
cranberry juice	stewed apricots	fresh apple w/cheese
roast bf (rare) corn on cob broccoli sprs. sliced orange salad stew. apples	veal steak spinach souff. strips raw crts. celery salad yogurt w/fruit	meat loaf honey glz. sqsh. caulif. w/cheese 2 pnapl. sl (diet) yogurt w/fruit
rye. brd./butr. milk, 8 oz. hot beverage	ww brd/butr. milk, 8 oz. hot beverage	rye brd./butr. milk, 8 oz. hot beverage
pl. gel. w/unswt. apple juice	frsh. fruit in season w/cheese	grape juice
turkey loaf veg. medley w/ parmesan chse. lettuce salad banana w/chse. grain brd/btr. milk, 8 oz. hot beverage	chkn. rice cass. grn. beans w/ onion/broc. bits mix. frsh. fruit salad pl. gel. w/grpe. ju. rye brd/btr. milk, 8 oz. hot beverage	pink roast lamb w/gravy esc. squash spec. cake toss. grn. salad stew. mix dried fruit ww brd./butter milk, 8 oz. hot beverage
yogurt[2] w/fruit	carrot juice	pl. gel. w/diet pears/lemon ju.

[1]Use only Certified (raw) milk, butter and cheese. DO NOT USE TOBACCO. Use only raw sugar or honey and fresh or frozen vegetables.
Read label of all ingredients, on all cans, bottles, boxes and packages to avoid foods with tomato sauce, tomato paste, paprika, red peppers, green peppers, eggplant, white potato flour and white potato starch.

[2]Economical brands may contain potato.

NUTRITIONAL DIET[1]

with ELIMINATION of Potato, Tomato, Peppers and Eggplant

WEDNESDAY	THURSDAY	FRIDAY	SATURDAY
stew. prunes granola buckwht. cakes w/honey, butter milk, 8 oz. hot beverage	half grapeft. ralston hard eggs crkwht. toast w/ btr., diet jelly milk, 8 oz. hot beverage	banana granola beef patty rye toast w/btr. diet jelly milk, 8 oz. hot beverage	orange juice oats poached egg ww toast w/btr. diet jelly milk, 8 oz. hot beverage
carrot juice	stewed apricots	grapefruit juice	carrot juice
baked chicken brown rice brussel sprouts pl. gel. w/cran. ju. & cot. cheese salad tangelos w/chse. spec. cookies grain brd./butr. milk, 8 oz. hot beverage	beef stew w/frsh. onion, peas & carrots toss. grn. salad yogurt w/fruit grape juice ww brd/butter milk, 8 oz. hot beverage	baked fish green beans mix. frsh. fruit salad pl. gel. w/frsh. orange slices grain brd./butr. milk, 8 oz. hot beverage	pink liver harvest beets mix. frsh. fruit salad yogurt w/fruit ww brd./butter milk, 8 oz. hot beverage
banana	prune juice	stewed apple	1 orange w/cheese
green pea soup cottage chse. & frsh. fruit plate spec. cookies yogurt/fruit rye brd/btr. milk, 8 oz. hot beverage	tstd. chse. sand. asparagus pl. gel. w/aplsce. salad baked apple w/cheese grain brd/btr. milk, 8 oz. hot beverage	diced beef w/ escal. corn peas & carrots frsh. grapes w/ cheese yogurt w/fruit rye brd/btr. milk, 8 oz. hot beverage	pink hamburger on rye bread frs. onion rings cole slaw pl. gel. w/banana rye brd./butter milk, 8 oz. hot beverage
apple juice	1 orange	carrot juice	lemon juice

Removing the Nightshade Toxins

Is it possible to remove the culprit toxins from the nightshades and make them acceptable to sensitive people? Research has not pinpointed all the chemicals in these crops. We think we know the critical ones but there could be others. As noted in Dr. Tso's Chapter V on Tobacco, 5000 chemicals already have been isolated and identified in tobacco and more are being named every month. Hence, the nightshades are complex and it likely would take years to identify most of the chemicals, then each would need to be tested on rats, perhaps people, to see if it is toxic. This would take time and money.

For years the potato breeders have been trying to keep the solanine in the hybrids below 20 mg/100 grams fresh weight of tubers. Solanine is relatively insoluble and varies in content with cultivars, as noted in Table 3. It takes a temperature of about 250°F to break it down.

Table 3. Fate of Glycoalkaloids Including Solanine in Cooked Potato Slices. (After Thomas Fitzpatrick, Eastern Regional Research Center, USDA, Phila., Pa. 19118).

Treatment of Slices	Potato Variety		
	Kennebec	Wauseon	Merrimac
	Solanine/100 grms Fresh Potato		
Fresh	15.0	7.53	8.52
Aged[1]	103.0	92.3	104.0
Aged Fried[2]	14.8	20.5	5.57
Aged microwaved	36.5	46.3	47.4
Aged Boiled	88.7	78.5	98.4
Water from Boil	14.3	----	----

[1]Incubated 5 days at room temperature.
[2]Deep fried in Crisco which contained no total glycoalkaloids on analysis after the frying.

It is apparent that frying the potatoes in hot grease significantly reduces the glycoalkaloids, including solanine, but for sensitive people, this is enough to induce aches and pains.

Substitute No-Nightshades Recipes

Linda LeBoeuf of Somerville, New Jersey, who along with her husband, Alan, is on the Childers' Diet, has prepared a number of No-Nightshades recipes that may be of interest. She has prepared a "Carato sauce" that tastes like a tomato sauce but has no tomatoes in it. We should note that some beets are included in her recipe and for some cooperators beets on successive days may result in aches. The amount of beets you get in these recipes, however, probably would not be a factor.

Incidentally, if you should develop an interesting and generally useful recipe, send it to us. We can repeat it for others to use in the next edition of this book with credit to you.

CARATO
(Substitute for Tomato)

4 lbs. fresh carrots
2 lemons
2 large fresh beets
1½ cups water

Cut carrots and beets into sections and cook in 1½ cups of water at high temperature in a covered pot for 10 minutes. If they are cooked enough you should be able to mash them with a potato masher until the color of the mash is a reddish orange. Squeeze in the two lemons and mash again. You now have enough "Caratoes" to make more than one of the following recipes.

Carato Sauce

6 cups Caratoes
½ cup parmesan cheese
¼ cup olive oil
2 tablespoons oregano
1 teaspoon basil
½ teaspoon black pepper
1 cup water
1 large onion chopped
Juice from 1 lemon
½ teaspoon salt
2 teaspoon garlic powder

Combine ingredients in large pot and cook at high temperature for ½ hour stirring frequently. Sauce may be thinned by adding water. Blend if smoother consistency is desired.

For meat sauce, first cook chopped meat in pot with chopped onions, then drain the fat. Then add the above ingredients and follow the same directions.

You will find "Carato" sauce a satisfactory sauce for any Italian recipe normally calling for tomato sauce, including lasagna, manicotti, or even pizza. Add meatballs.

Chili Con Carne

2 lbs. ground beef
3 cups Carato sauce
2 tablespoons horseradish
1 tablespoon black pepper
4 onions chopped
2 cans kidney beans with liquid (15½ ounces)

Cook ground beef and onions in deep fry pan until brown. Drain off fat. Stir in Caratoes, kidney beans and seasonings. Heat to boil. Reduce heat, simmer ½ hour. Serves 10.

Manhattan Clam Chowder

2-6 ounce cans whole baby clams in salt water
1 cup Caratoes
¼ cup chopped celery
½ cup thinly sliced leeks
1½ teaspoons thyme
4 whole cloves
1 teaspoon freshly ground black pepper
2 cans hominy (liquid drained)
4 cups water
¼ cup Carato catsup
¼ cup chopped parsley
½ cup chopped onion
1 bay leaf crumbled
2 teaspoons salt
clove garlic

Combine ingredients. Bring to a boil. Reduce heat and simmer for 20 minutes. Serves 6.

New England Clam Chowder

2-6 ounce cans whole baby clams in salt water
4 cups milk, scalded
3 tablespoons butter
2 bay leaves crumbled
3-12 ounce cans hominy (liquid drained)
1½ cups onions, chopped
2 tablespoons flour

Combine ingredients and simmer for 30 minutes; add freshly ground black pepper to taste.

French Dressing

⅔ cup olive oil
½ cup Caratoes
½ teaspoon prepared mustard
½ cup red wine vinegar
¼ cup orange juice
¼ teaspoon garlic powder

Combine ingredients in blender and blend for 30 seconds at high speed.

Russian Dressing

½ cup Caratoes
1 tablespoon chopped green olives (pimentoes removed)
½ cup mayonnaise
1 teaspoon snipped chives
½ teaspoon horseradish

Combine ingredients in bowl. Blend thoroughly with a spoon. Salt and pepper to taste.

Catsup

1 cup Caratoes
2 tablespoons water
½ teaspoon salt
5 tablespoons vinegar
1 tablespoon sugar or honey
¼ teaspoon onion powder

Combine all ingredients in blender and blend at low speed for 60 seconds.

Bloody Mary Mix

¾ cup Caratoes
1 lemon squeezed
⅓ cup water
1 tablespoon horseradish

Combine ingredients in blender and blend at low speed for 60 seconds. Salt and pepper to taste.

POTATO SUBSTITUTES

Mashed Chick Peas
(Mashed potato substitute)

2-12 ounce cans of chick peas

Drain liquid from cans. Shell each pea before placing it in a pot with ½ cup of water. Heat peas then drain water. Mash the peas until they have the same consistency as mashed potatoes. Add milk to soften if you like. Serve with butter or gravy. These chick peas can also be whipped for a smoother consistency. Serves 4 or 5.

Home Fries

2 large sweet potatoes sliced   1 large onion diced
2 tablespoon butter

Melt butter in fry pan. Add onion then potatoes. Cook until brown and soft. Serves four.

NOTE: Rice Fryes are available in some market places.

What Doctors are Prescribing

The Arthritis Foundation has distributed the following information on drugs being prescribed by doctors for relief from arthritis. Drugs give only temporary relief and nearly all are harmful to the body in one way or another. Some have serious side effects.

If you are on the No-Nightshades Diet, it would be well to gradually reduce, then stop any drugs you may be taking unless for some serious reason it is mandatory that you continue. The human body was not made to need drugs regularly. Rather than continuing to treat the symptoms, let's get at the basic cause and correct it.

There are a number of paperbacks in book stores and libraries on prescription drugs, giving their generic names, when prescribed, warnings, precautions, side effects and adverse reactions. If you are taking a drug regularly, you may wish to acquaint yourself with its pros and cons. One such booklet is E.L. Stern's "Your Guide to Prescription Drugs" Grosset and Dunlap, New York. 80pp. 1975. A professional book is "Modern Drug Encyclopedia — A Compendium" by A. J. Lewis et al., Editors, Yorke Medical Books, 666 5th Ave., New York, N.Y. 1979. 1056 pp.

CORTISONE (STEROIDS®)

Used in Treating: Systemic Lupus Erythematosus, Rheumatoid Arthritis, Juvenile Rheumatoid Arthritis, Dermatomyositis, Polymyositis, Vasculitis.

Q. What is Cortisone and how does it work?

A. Cortisone or Hydrocortisone are generic terms which apply to a vast number of drugs which contain corticosteroids (often referred to as steroids). Prednisone is the type of steroid used most frequently in treating the systemic rheumatic diseases. Cortisone has been shown to reduce the signs and symptoms of the above diseases by reducing swelling, relieving pain and duration of morning stiffness, and providing increased mobility.

Q. Is Cortisone always effective in every patient who takes it?

A. No. However, Cortisone carries with it the risk of serious side effects so that your physician will consider very seriously your disease activity before prescribing Cortisone.

Q. What are the side effects of Cortisone?

A. There are many side effects to Cortisone therapy. The one patients will notice first is fluid retention, which results in a weight gain. Individuals on Cortisone therapy might also notice easy bruising of the skin. Other side effects include peptic ulcer, cataracts, obesity, sugar diabetes and acne. Other serious hazards of Cortisone therapy are infections and bone fractions. All patients on Cortisone should carry identification that they are on that drug, as doctors in an emergency room must give more Cortisone should a patient be in a serious accident, or develop another life-threatening disease. More Cortisone must also be given prior to an operation. If you notice any uncommon effects while taking Cortisone, report them immediately to your physician.

Q. Should I stop taking Cortisone if I experience side effects?

A. No. Your physician must work with you on discontinuing Cortisone therapy. Usually he will begin to decrease your dosage gradually but not stop it immediately. Decreasing the dosage of Cortisone must usually be done gradually in order to avoid adrenal failure (diarrhea, low blood pressure, fainting).

Q. How is Cortisone administered?

A. Most of the time, Cortisone will be prescribed as a pill to be taken by mouth. However, occasional injections of Cortisone directly into an affected joint provide temporary relief. One will not interfere with the other, and patients who receive occasional joint injections will not need to interrupt their oral dosage. Sometimes Cortisone is given by another route as in the treatment of eye disease with eye drops.

Q. Can Cortisone be taken with other arthritis medication?

A. Yes. Cortisone is often given in conjunction with gold, aspirin, indomethacin and immunosuppressives. It is advisable to tell your physician of any medications you are taking that have not been prescribed by him, including those which you have purchased over the counter.

HYDROXYCHLOROQUINE (PLAQUENIL®)

Used in Treating: Systemic Lupus Erythematosus (SLE) and Rheumatoid Arthritis (RA).

Q. What is Hydroxychloroquine and how does it work?

A. Hydroxychloroquine is an antimalarial drug. It has been shown to decrease the signs and symptoms of rheumatoid arthritis by reducing joint swelling and providing increased mobility and decreasing the extent and severity of the rash in SLE. It is sometimes used in patients with RA who have not responded to gold therapy or in others as combined treatment with aspirin. Hydroxychloroquine does not provide a response immediately and often patients will not notice improvement for several weeks and maximum benefit may take several months.

Q. Can any patient with rheumatoid arthritis or SLE receive Hydroxychloroquine?

A. No. Your physician will decide if and when you might be started on Hydroxychloroquine (antimalarial therapy) based on examination and laboratory findings.

Q. Is Hydroxychloroquine effective in every patient who takes it?

A. No. Which is why you must continue to see your physician. He must design a treatment program that is right for you.

Q. What are the side effects of Hydroxychloroquine?

A. The most common side effects are skin rash and keratitis (deposits in the eye). More serious problems with the eyes may also occur which can lead to blindness and your physician will ask you to have periodic eye examinations by an ophthalmologist. If you experience these or other effects while taking Hydroxychloroquine, report them immediately to your physician.

Q. Should I stop taking Hydroxychloroquine if I experience side effects?

A. Yes, but it is not wise to discontinue any medication without first talking with your physician and getting his approval to do so. What you are experiencing may not be a result of the Hydroxychloroquine.

Q. How is Hydroxychloroquine administered?

A. Hydroxychloroquine is a prescription drug supplied in tablets to be taken by mouth. It is a cumulative drug, which means that you should not expect immediate response because Hydroxychloroquine must accumulate in our system before benefit can be obtained. Minimum response can occur in several weeks but for a maximum effect, the drug must accumulate for several months.

Q. Can Hydroxychloroquine be taken with other arthritis medication?

A. Yes. Hydroxychloroquine is often given in conjunction with salicylates (aspirin) and steroids (cortisone). It is advisable to tell your physician of any medication you are taking not prescribed by him, including those which you have purchased over the counter.

PHENYLBUTAZONE (BUTAZOLIDIN®)

Used in Treating: Gouty Arthritis, Ankylosing Spondylitis, and other Rheumatic Diseases such as Bursitis, Fibrositis, Tendinitis, and Fasciitis.

Q. What is Phenylabutazone and what does it do?

A. Phenylbutazone is a nonsteroidal anti-inflammatory agent. That is to say, it is a drug which *contains no cortisone,* but acts to fight the inflammation of arthritis. Phenybutazone has been found to be effective in relieving pain and reduce swelling, morning stiffness and disease activity.

Q. Can anyone with gout, spondylitis or the other mentioned diseases take Phenylbutazone?

A. No. It will depend upon each individual's disease activity and involvement. Phenylabutazone has undesirable side effects and your physician must assess each case individually.

Q. What are the side effects to Phenylbutazone?

A. The most serious side effects is bone marrow depression. Other side effects include fluid retention which can result in weight gain, rash, peptic ulceration, and liver damage. Your physician will perform frequent laboratory tests so these can be avoided.

Q. Should I stop taking Phenylbutazone if side effects occur?

A. Yes, but it is not wise to discontinue the drug on your own. Your physician will be watching you closely for side effects and he can make a judgment as to whether you should or should not discontinue the drug.

Q. How is Phenylbutazone administered?

A. Phenylbutazone is a prescription drug supplied in tablets to be taken by mouth.

Q. Can I take Phenylbutazone with other arthritis medication?

A. Phenylbutazone can be given in conjunction with other arthritis medication such as gold and steriods (cortisone). It is advisable to tell your physician of any medication you may be taking, not prescribed by him including those which you have purchased over the counter.

All You Need To

Do Is To Go Back

To The Nightshades

And Your Miseries Will

Be Refunded!

CHAPTER III

Case Histories, Comments

Letters From Cooperators

Following letters have been received from cooperators since the first edition of this book in October 1977. The headings for each letter will help you find responses that apply to your particular case. Letters are typical of hundreds received, totalling well over 18,000 since the start of tests in 1975. Cooperators total about 3000 at printing of this edition, of which about 72% are showing various degrees of positive response, varying from obvious to miraculous. Where cooperators are not getting a positive response, totalling about 28%, this is believed to be due to (a) not really being on the Diet, (b) over-medication, (c) not understanding the diet from the outset, (d) not really wanting to give up these foods in the first place, (e) an overshadowing of other health problems, or (f) not staying with the Diet long enough to get results based on their initial condition. Where we have had local contact and guidance with cooperators, and they are rigidly on the Diet, we have yet to see anyone who has not responded positively and many of them markedly.

The files of these letters are open to responsible researchers who may wish to study correlations or contribute to our knowledge of how the nightshades are affecting human health.

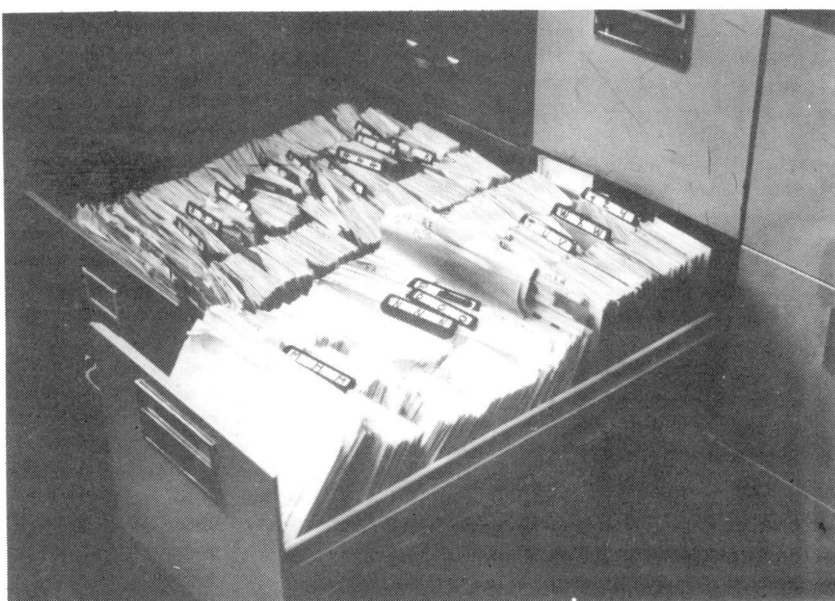

Figure 1. Each envelope in these files contains correspondence from one of over 3000 cooperators on the *Childers' No-Nightshades Diet.* These cooperators are located around the world, but mostly in the USA and Canada.

IT IS A MIRACLE

I am 50, 140 lbs., have had severe arthritic problems for only 2 yrs. with a frozen right shoulder joint, aching spine, other joints, tendinitis in knees, hands, hips, shoulders, neck and back. All symptoms stopped and moles stopped growing within only one month after eliminating the nightshades. I was consuming all these foods every day of the week, except eggplant. I had been treated with cortisone joint injections, butazolidin and anti-inflammation drugs. Now I can do all my work without pain or crippling effect — it is a miracle! I have told others with symptoms like mine but some are very skeptical, won't try it and still hurt. A few others said it helped them. It is amazing how many of the prepared foods contain some form of the nightshades. Why has your discovery not received world-wide acclaim? My right shoulder had become completely frozen and it regained complete movement. Now I am apparently totally healed and feel strong again. Thank you, thank you. EAF:Ga.

MADE A MEAL OF TOMATOES AND GREEN PEPPERS

I read an article on your Diet to my brother who has stiffness and aches and pains badly. He thought it was due to cultivating and work with his farm crops. But he was making a meal out of tomatoes and green peppers. He loves them. He completely stopped these foods, all nightshades, and in a matter of days he was greatly relieved of aches and pains. He is a real believer in what you say and dodges the nightshades every day now.JS:MO.

I CAN WEAR MY RINGS AGAIN!

We have been on the No-Nightshades diet for about 4 mos. and I do have considerably better use of my hands. I can take lecture notes again in long-hand at conferences. In fact, the quality of my hand writing is much improved. Of little consequence to anyone but me, is the fact that I now can wear some of my favorite rings which I had put away "forever." Disfigurement in my hands seems to have improved a little.

As for John, he checks regularly with the arthritis specialist at Hahnemann Medical School and they find no further deterioration. In fact, the knee that had to be drained has needed no further attention. John is back on his bicycle and does four long laps a day around town. He looks a lot better and has much more pep. (Over 80 yrs.). M&JC:N.J.

CAN SCRATCH MY BACK AGAIN!

Following your advice on the No-Nightshades diet means that I can once again take off my coat and scratch my back without pain. Also, it means a good nights rest without waking up several times because of pains in my legs and shoulders. It really works! Once in awhile I get a recurrence and when I read the label on the can of soup I have eaten, there it is — one of the nightshades among the ingredients. No more aspirin, and I used to take at least 6 a day.It's wonderful. I do again thank you. NB:N.Y.

NOW — A FEELING OF WELL BEING!

It has been 9 months since I began to eliminate the nightshades from my diet. My arthritis has shown continuous improvement. First the muscles felt better, less and less stiffness and pain, more and more ease of movement, less clumsiness, but my hand writing has not improved much yet. Next, the joints in my hands, shoulders, neck, and hips lost the pain. The hands, where the arthritis first began, continued to experience an occasional twinge, usually related to something I inadvertently ate. But now the pain of all these joints is gone most of the time. I can even sleep on my stomach once more, now that I can turn my neck to the side and stand pressure. Overall, I have noticed a general feeling of well being that stays with me. For years I have been moody and felt depressed a good part of the time for no reason that I could detect. Now it feels quite natural to be "up" and positive. This has been an unexpected benefit and has continued for the nine months, which eliminates the possibility of a fluke.

In general, I have less trouble with allergies. I have had sinusitis and much sneezing for years and have needed heavy medication with demitane, particularly during pollination season. I now need only one pill at night and none in the morning. Also, a continuous soreness in my lower abdominal region, which has plagued me for years, is gone. I seem to be able to eat anything (except the nightshades) with impunity.

There has been only one problem and your Newscard recently gave me the clue. I started losing weight with the Nutrilite Weight Control Plan but my thumb after awhile got sore as I began to ingest the food supplements. I quit these and now I am back to normal with no soreness. How wonderful it is to understand what is happening and to realize that I have options I hadn't dreamed of years ago. Along with my arthritis, my fingernails had become full of ridges. Now they are smooth.

Although I am constantly telling people about the Diet, there have been few takers and I can understand this. Most people have severe doubts, can't think of giving up their favorite foods, and are willing to go along with pain that doesn't apparently hurt enough yet, rather than take the challenge of change. I deal with this constantly. Within the past year, with such energy and a happier view of life, I have taken and passed the California exam for Marriage, Family and Child Counselling and have started a private practice. Sometimes I feel as if I have a new body and, certainly, I have a new life.

May I contribute some money to your research? How do I do it? ERP:Ca.

Note: This lady is 56 yrs., weighs 135 lbs., was eating potatoes, tomatoes and peppers a few times a wk., had colitis, hadn't smoked for 25 yrs., and had had (diagnosed) arthritis for about 5 yrs.

"DRUNK-LIKE" AND GROPING

I could not walk up the stairs without hanging onto the banister. Left shoulder and right toes ached all the time. I was drunkish and groping in a stupor and I don't drink. My main diet had been tomato, eggplant, potatoes and peppers. I also canned them. All symptoms have disappeared since eliminating the nightshades. Bless you! MR:N.J.

TIRED ALL MY LIFE

I read about your Diet in many magazines. Also, a friend told me to cut out the nightshades so last May I did (now, following April). At start, my shoulder was very stiff and I have always had a lot of allergies. My shoulder is now loose — no problem, and I am not tired any more. I used to say I was born tired. Evidently my body has been battling the nightshades all my life. As a child I was "allergic" to eggplant, rhubarb, radishes and peppers and I had to use gloves to peel an orange or my skin would crack around the nails. Now my sinus is okay; it bothered me for years. I just went through 9 days of cold wet weather and felt fine the whole time. MAN:Ca.

Note: This lady is 70 yrs., had problems 49 yrs., 145 lbs., radical mastectomy (left) 30 yrs. ago, gall bladder surgery 9 yrs. ago and many moles all her life. NFC

BLOOD TESTS OK NOW

I am 54, 148 lbs. (on a diet now), have had increasing aches and pains the past year, taking motrin, iron, exercising as much as I can. I have been on the No-Nightshades Diet about 2 yrs. and whereas my sediment blood count was high at the start I was told, the doctor now says my rheumatoid arthritis is under control with a low sediment count. I can't drink coffee at all — it makes me tremble; tea seems okay. I am enthusiastic supporter of your work and have told many people. FLK:N.J.

RHEUMATOID ARTHRITIS, DEGENERATIVE SPINAL DISEASE

I am 50 years, have had the problems for 20 years in feet, back, hands, hips, elbows, shoulders and neck very badly with lighter problem in ankles, knees and chest, have taken indocin and butazolidin pills, ate nightshades regularly and in quantity sometimes. I have been on your Diet for 6 months. Ninety percent of the pain has left, was retired 6 years ago with rheumatoid arthritis and degenerative spinal disease. I have several other people in this area on the Diet which has worked well for them too." G.B.S., NM

TOOK FIVE MONTHS

"I had no relief from the Diet until the fifth month. In the 6th month I have over 75% relief from arthritis and tendinitis. If relief continues, I should be free of pain in a year." C.S.:Ind.

MUST BE YOUR OWN DETECTIVE

(Letter to Dr. Carleton Fredericks, Nutritionist, Radio Station WOR, New York City)

"I am a 28-yr. old female. Three years ago I became severely ill with arthritis of the spine, urinary tract infection, and a severe conjunctivitis in both eyes. After being ill for over 4 months and going from doctor to doctor, a New York City rheumatologist diagnosed me as having a disease called Reiter's Syndrome, an unusual form of arthritis that strikes young people and is rare in women.

"After the acute onset of the disease I continued to have joint pain which badly affected my spine (it was thought I may have Ankylosing Spondylitis, rare in women), knees, feet, ankles, hips, neck, and jaw joint.

"I went off and on medication (aspirin, Indocin, Clinoril, cortisone shots, etc.) as the pain and flare-ups continued. I was feeling very depressed and quite hopeless from being sick so much of the time. In looking back, I was growing a garden in summers and eating tomatoes, peppers and eggplant like a manaic.

"In December of 1978 I heard about the "No-Nightshades" Diet at which point I was so miserable that I was ready to try anything.

"After being on the Diet for three months I started to feel better, not knowing whether to attribute my improvement to the Diet or, and I quote the Arthritis Foundation, "The natural remission of arthritis", I decided to go off the Diet and test it. That night after eating some tomato and pepper products I became sick, so sick that I thought a truck had run over me. Several of my affected joints were very painful.

"I have been strictly on the Diet ever since and have slowly continued to improve. Right now I am at least 60% improved. It is a beautiful and safe way to control the pain of arthritis. I once again feel like a human being.

"Dr. Childers has called my home a few times over the past year to help me with the Diet, and for that I am very grateful. It is not a simple diet. There are many pitfalls, the worst of which is not really understandig the Diet at the outset, thinking you are on it, then saying that it did not work. The nightshades are hidden in so many foods that you really have to be your own detective. A small amount of them, as a bit of paprika or potato starch in my system, is enough to keep the problem going.

"I hope Dr. Childers receives the recognition that he so rightly deserves, the reason I am writing you with so many listeners. He is a dedicated and caring man who has discovered a million dollar idea that does not cost even a penny to do."

"I also hope that some of the seemingly biased doctors will soon learn about this Diet approach to arthritis and begin to suggest it to their patients as a part of a program to get them well. The "No-Nightshades" Diet for the control of arthritis is a powerful story that must be told." RS:N.J.

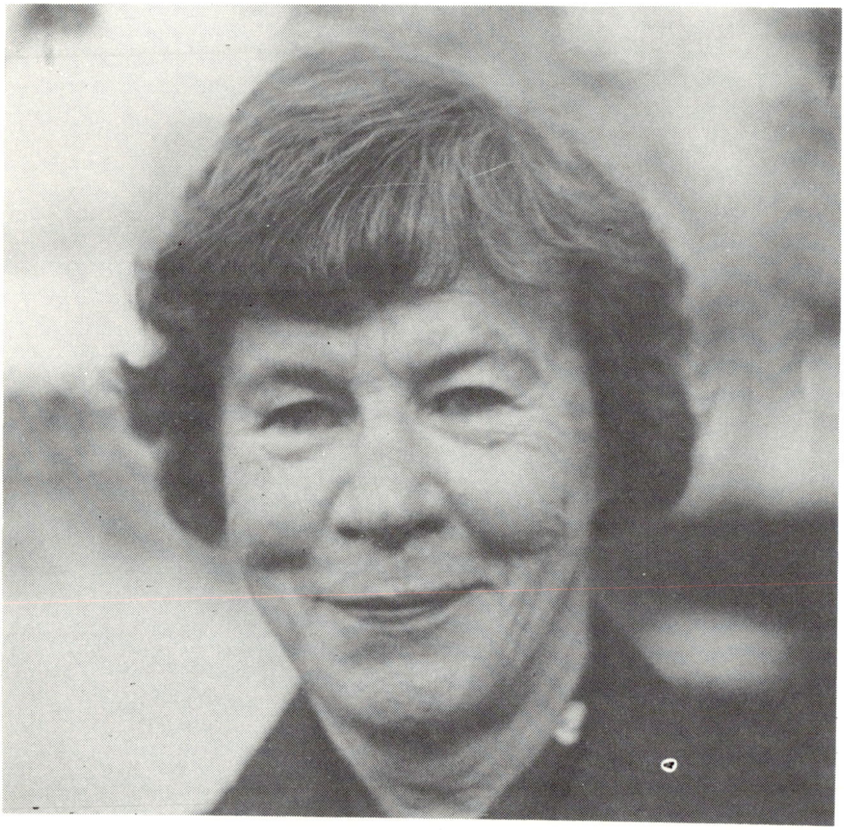

Mrs. Alma P. Hough, a career woman, of Somerville, New Jersey, thinking of retiring, was among the first to try the Diet in 1975. She recovered completely from aches and pains in the knees, feet, shoulder, lower abdomen, hands and wrist which had been broken. Five years later she was anxious to keep working eight hours a day as Advertising Manager for a local newspaper. (Photo by Messenger-Gazette, Somerville, N.J.)

A LETTER TO CONSUMER REPORTS

To: Consumer Reports, 256 Washington St., Mt. Vernon, NY 10550

"I note in a recent issue of Consumer Reports that one of the books not recommended to arthritic patients is the book "Nightshades and Health" by Norman F. Childers and Gerard M. Russo.

In view of my own experience and several people around me, I feel compelled to write to you. In July, 1975, I went on Dr. Childers' "No Nightshades" Diet. For several years I had suffered arthritis of the knee, wrist and a constant problem of the pelvic area, where I had had surgery 20 years previous. Within three months all of these problems had disappeared. And again, my "new" nimble fingers could deal cards at our bridge club. After several months on the diet, I decided to resume eating the nightshades, white potato, red and green peppers, eggplant and tomatoes. I do not use tobacco. In about ten days all of my problems returned. Returning to the "No Nightshades" Diet required almost two weeks for my ailments to disappear. Since that time I have adhered strictly to the diet and I am without any of the previous pain and ailments for which I had repeatedly, and unsuccessfully, sought medical help.

I believe that I can speak for dozens of others in this area who have shown marked improvement or complete recovery on the Diet. Many of the public libraries in North Jersey carry Dr. Childers' book and they report a long waiting list.

I am one of thousands of cooperators in this country and around the world who report back to Dr. Childers. He has been issuing periodic newsletters and reports of recent findings, all free, I might add. I am in contact with many of his cooperators and I have heard of nothing but success by former arthritis sufferers.

In the Arthritis Foundation's rejection of Dr. Childers' book and others, it neglected to put forth any scientific reason. How do they REVIEW the books? Is it on the basis of scientific research? How much research have they done on Dr. Childers' diet?

It puzzles me to note that the medical profession continues to adhere to drugs and surgery as the cornerstone of arthritis treatment when so many of the drugs have disastrous side effects and, in the end, only kill the pain while the problems worsen.

I hope for the good of so many arthritis victims that both Consumer Reports and The Arthritis Foundation will do a more thorough scientific study before making, what to me, is an erroneous assumption." Alma P. Hough, Somerville, N.J.

ANGINA PECTORIS CLEARED!

"On the nightshades Diet my *Angina pectoris* has disappeared. "Cardiac Arrhythmias" a book edited by Dreifus and Likoff states that "atropine, the active ingredient in belladonna (a nightshade), accelerates the heart beat, as recorded by the AV-model pacemaker, setting the stage for *Angina*." R.L.T.:NJ

LETTER TO ROBERT RODALE, ORGANIC GARDENING MAGAZINE

"At mid-life I developed a sudden sensitivity to the alkaloids contained in nightshade plants — tomatoes, potatoes, peppers — the vegetable staples of my diet! The symptoms are so much like arthritis that I did not question it, I simply believed I was coming down with crippling arthritis. Within two years my hands were unable to grip the steering wheel to drive. Hip joints ached when I walked, especially uphill. Right shoulder became inflamed and froze painfully after a day of scything weeds. Neck and spine ached so badly that I was unable to pick a row of beans without stopping to rest every few feet. I was certain that I would soon become unable to continue any activity. Then I read an article in the August '78 issue of Organic Gardening about how the alkaloids in nightshades cause arthritis-like symptoms in some sensitive people, and the research being done on this by Dr. Norman Childers of Rutgers University. The article described exactly what was happening to me! I immediately eliminated all nightshades from my diet and within two weeks the pain in my joints was gone. On a strict no-nightshades diet my joints appear to be healing; my strength has returned, health has been restored to me. It is truly a miracle. I am so grateful! Thank you for publishing that article. I wish everyone who thinks they have arthritis could read it. From now on my garden will grow lots of greens, beans, peas, and delicious members of the cole. family, and I won't miss those nightshades at all!" E.A.F., GA.

PERSONALTY CHANGE

My mother went on your Diet last summer and within a few months her personality has changed completely from depressed, hypersensitive (taking pills for these problems), and withdrawn. Now she is outward, not frantic about things, happy and steady in her outlook. I am her daughter and have had the same problems with similar recovery. We just wanted you to know this for your research program. Arthritis is "not" a problem with us — yet! AS:N.J.

DON'T NEED GLASSES FOR DRIVING ANY MORE

I am 62, 175 lbs., been on your Diet for about 6 mos. after reading about it in the local Chicago paper. I have been feeling exceptionally well and was amazed recently to notice an improvement in my vision. I usually wear glasses for distance viewing while driving, but I did not need them. Your research and discovery have made a tremendous difference in my life and I want to thank you. I have a large mole on my back but no difference in size or appearance as yet. *(Note: with several other cooperators, we have found that after 5 yrs. strictly on the diet, these moles will lose their rugged caps and gradually shrink in size. Smaller moles will disappear with only a dark level spot left. We know that moles are watched for cancer development. NFC).* Here is $25 for a book. Keep the change. WHH:Il.

QUACK DEVICES!

Note: Following is a rather typical comment from syndicated doctors answering letters from their fans. Item appeared in Express News, San Antonio, Tx. Cooperators send many of these to us. Lawrence E. Lamb, MD, is the doctor. NFC.

Q. Do the people sending me the enclosed brochure of a book on nightshades know what they are talking about. Will the diet really help me?

A. Regardless of what value the book described in the folder might have from a horticultural point of view, I don't believe that these will be of any help at all for arthritics. The nightshades include such *diverse* plants as potatoes, tomatoes, peppers and eggplant. *(Note: they belong to the same plant family).* These foods do not cause arthritis. Eliminating them from your diet will not cure arthritis. Unfortunately, there are multiple quack devices to obtain money from sufferers of arthritis. I wish we had a more effective means of protecting the public from misinformation. The presence of a free press makes it very difficult to do this and, of course, a free press is important to us. As a general rule, I would say do not subscribe to any treatment that is offered to you through the mail or at your door. Don't buy "magic" medicines or use products that are advertised to cure your arthritis in public magazines. Consult your doctor or with a severe case of arthritis see a rheumatoid specialist. Send 50¢ and we can send you "Osteoarthritis; Degeneratuve or wear and tear arthritis."

MYASTHENIA GRAVIS?

MG is another form of arthritis (fatal to Mr. Onassis, Greek shipping magnet and husband of Jackie Kennedy Onassis). A lady in her 70's in Florida was suddenly taken sick with this disease, *Myasthenia gravis,* as medically diagnosed, and was in a wheelchair for awhile. There were severe leg pains and muscle weakness, being able to lift her leg only a few inches while laying in bed. Use of 60 mg of mestinon every three hours enabled her to use a walker. Usually with MG there is not much pain but this lady had considerable pain and the M.D. diagnosed this part as arthritis but the question arose as to where one disease started and the other stopped. There appears to be some confusion among doctors. She had been on the Adele Davis' diet from her book, "Let's Get Well", but had seen little appreciable change and was still taking mestinon 7-8 hours/day. Then suddenly after several weeks on the "No-Nightshades" Diet she started getting better and later was diagnosed in John Hopkins Hospital in Baltimore, Md. as "having no evidence of MG". A remission? She is still confused as to whether the Davis' or No-Nightshades' Diet was effective but will not take a chance on partaking of the nightshades for fear of recurrence of MG. *(Note: Dr. Carleton Fredericks of WOR Station, NYC, believes there is a chance that glaucoma may respond to the Diet since these two diseases are related.) G.S.:Fla. Late Note: She started eating tomatoes again; leg pains returned!*

PAPRIKA IS THE SNEAKY SINNER!

I am 64, 160 lbs, eating potatoes and tomatoes regularly, and have had arthritic problems for 20 yrs in my feet, ankles, knees, hands, hips elbows, shoulders, chest, neck and back. I have had stomach cramps often. I walk a lot and take mild pain killers with some Regroton when blood pressure is up. I started the Diet Labor Day and it is four weeks later. Already the stiffness is leaving my joints, especially my neck. I can feel the pain leaving all over except in my right shoulder which has been the worst from the beginning of my arthritis. Almost a year later I must say the improvement I have had from the Diet is indescribable. Only problem is invitations to dinner of which I am accepting less and less. I have my company here at home. I simply cannot believe the improvement I have made. I take back all I said about the book not being worth the money! My husband has improved but not as much as I; at least he does not take ascription anymore. He was taking 6 a day. I can always tell when I get into paprika — it is in so many things I find that are not even labelled. It is the sneaky little sinner. Thanks a million for the relief we have gotten. AR:Fla.; Panama City.

CANCER AND THE TOBACCO NIGHTSHADE

While working in So. Calif. as a waiter in 1963, it was mandatory to carry a food handlers card and a chest X-ray was required. Later that year I moved to Phoenix, Arizona where another X-ray was demanded and this one showed a spot on my left lung. I was okeyed and there seemed no cause for alarm. I had been trying to stop smoking but with little success. Then about that time the first Surgeon General's Report appeared on smoking and lung cancer and this scared me to the point of quitting cigarettes in late 1964. This was no small feat since I was at least a 2-pack/day smoker. Again in 1968-9 the X-ray showed the spot and the doctor said no cause for alarm but there was no guarantee. In 1973 my left kidney was removed because of cancer and in late 1973 I had the left lobe of my lung removed. There is no doubt in my mind that had I NOT stopped smoking when I did, I would not be writing this letter. Stopping smoking was the best favor I ever did for myself.

I am strictly on the No-Nightshades Diet now, no cancer 7 yrs later, and feel fine but my wife is not convinced of its merits. FO:N.J.

PICKLED HERRING, MATZAH, PASSOVER FOODS — NO, NOS!

Before reading your article in the Philadelphia Evening Bulletin, I was eating potatoes, tomatoes and peppers daily; eggplant, paprika and pizza occasionally. Happy to tell you I am a new person since I gave them up. I can open and close faucets, open and shut windows, and button blouses. Pickled herring, Passover foods, and Matzah especially are on my No No list. With admiration and appreciation, I thank you. Hope you are well and enjoying a pleasant summer too. GR:N.J.

A REVIEW OF "THE NIGHTSHADES AND HEALTH" BOOK AND REPLY.

Note: The following book review and reply appeared in HortScience, a publication of the American Society for Hortcultural Science, Vol. 13, No. 2, 207-8. 1978. There are over 4000 professional members of this Society over the world. The review was made by an analytical chemist in food science, initially from Norway, and now at Purdue University, Lafayette, Indiana, a leading state in tomato production, processing and marketing.

The art of cooking is often confused with a process whereby a number of ingredients — a pinch of this, a dab of that, are thrown into the pot, boiled, and stirred with hopes that a delicious concoction will ensue. To experienced cooks it is obvious that such an attitude often ends in disaster. This process if applied to other human endeavours, such as book writing, will also have a similar unhappy ending. We know that careful consideration has to be given to the kind and quality of the ingredients, their balance and compatibility, and the sequence and methods of incorporation.

None of these basic principals have been followed by the authors of this book. Take a look at the ingredients: 1) Lengthy transcripts from the *Congressional Record* testifying to the excellence and utility of agricultural research (p 8-14); 2) description of a nightshade-free diet which in addition to preventing rheumatic and arthritic troubles is claimed to cure skin rash, thinning of the blood, tennis elbow, tender nipples and a host of other ailments (p 18-26); 3) testimonies by letter from some 80 collaborators (patients?), (in addition to the senior author) of alleged improvements of ailments after switching to the diet (p 27-39); 4) a learned discussion, by A. Zitnak, of the glycoalkaloids of nightshades (they are not found in tomato fruit and eggplant) (p 41-92); 5) a review by T. C. Tso of the production and composition of tobacco and tobacco smoke, the ill effects of smoking, and possible beneficial by-products of tobacco production (fraction I Protein) (p 93-121); 6) a short review by G. K. Davis of a disease affecting calcium metabolism in Argentine livestock when consuming a local pasture nightshade, profusely illustrated with photographs of viscera and muscle (p 123-136); 7) a collection of abstracts dealing with noxious substances in plants and including such diverse subjects as legumes, locoweed, oxaltes in forages, serum transaminase, Colorado beetles, lupin alkaloids, hypersensitivity etc., etc. (p 137-168; 8) a list of some common toxic plants (p 169-181).

The resulting concoction is rendered even more indigestible when it is suggested that the incidence of stomach cancer is related to the growing of nightshades in the backyard. The senior author's intention in publishing this book is apparently to convince the reader that the causative agents of a number of degenerative diseases are to be found in the nightshades and that a cure is possible by removing these from the diet. Unfortunately, he did not succeed with this reviewer. The morass of evidence is just too incoherent, nonsensical, and flamboyantly unscientific to be taken seriously.

Johan E. Hoff
Purdue University

NOTE: The following reply to the above review was given by Dr. A. H. Thompson, University of Maryland, College Park. He also is the author of the letter following this one. He repeats some of his experiences here but he also gives other opinions regarding the need for more research in the nightshades and health area from a scientific viewpoint. NFC.

Norman Childers' new book, *The Nightshades and Health,* is being received with alarm in some horticultural departments across the land, and with some most unscientific responses in others. Coming from scientists I find this difficult to understand, for I am one of his several hundred cooperators who is now living evidence that Norman Childers has indeed discovered something.

I have been deteriorating physically for 20 years with arthritis of the lower spine. All I have ever been able to get from medical science for this devastating disorder is the aspirin tablet and this is no weapon at all for the struggle against increasing odds. Life to me in 1976 became so restricted, so painful, and so useless that I decided I had to retire in the spring of 1978 when I would reach a natural stopping point in my responsibilities to graduate students.

A chance booking with Norman Childers on an airliner last spring led to the chance disclosure of his connection between arthritis and natural toxins (presumably alkaloids) found in members of the nightshade family. His evidence was so remarkable that I eliminated the nightshades from my diet immediately, but I did so without conviction, with some desperation perhaps, and with utterly nothing to lose. One by one painful daily realities disappeared from my world as spring unfolded. For a long time I could not believe what was happening to me — and did not. It simply couldn't be that easy.

But it was. Incredibly by mid-June I was back to normal, painless, daily activity I thought was gone forever for me. I could get out of bed or a chair normally; I could bend over and tie my own shoelaces again; I could get down to measure a fruit tree trunk circumference again — something I had not done in this decade. In just three months the pain and restricted movement from 20 years of arthritis was gone! And it happened without a *single aspirin; I simply had eliminated the Solanaceae* from my diet. Even today I find it all quite amazing.

The reaction is apparently reversible. At Dr. Childers' suggestion I went back to the *Solanaceae* for a week in July. Potato salad and fresh tomatoes are favorite foods, and I made the most of the respite. But I paid

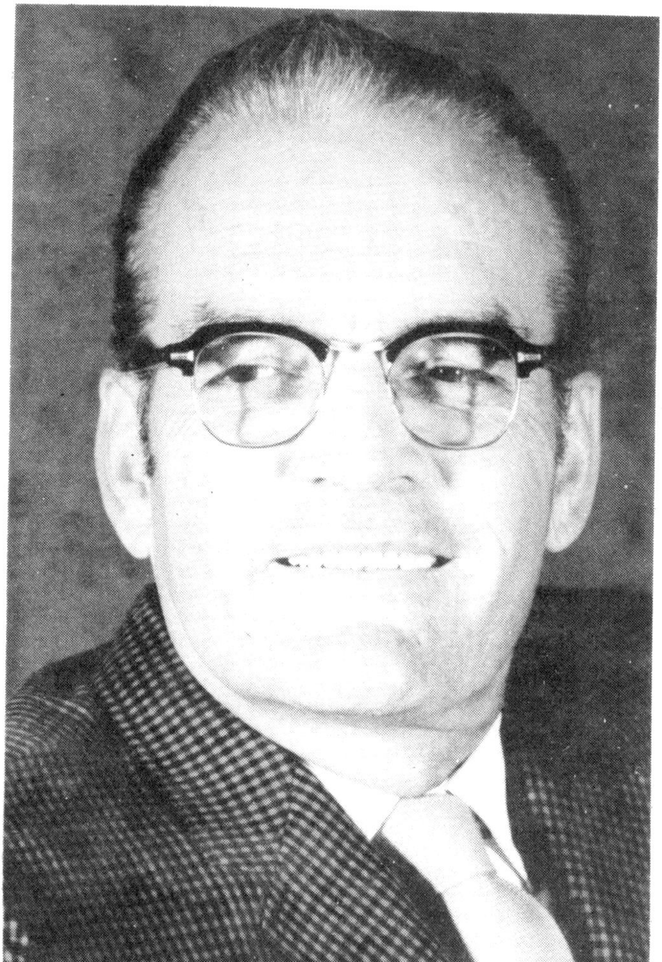

Dr. Arthur H. Thompson
University of Maryland, College Park.
"I find it all quite amazing. I was going to retire early.

my dues for that week with the old familiar back pains, a mild situation which took about two weeks to correct.

In recent years we in horticulture have felt unjustly persecuted at times with insults from EPA, environmentalists, organized labor, etc. We have reacted defensively to meet these challenges one way or another. Now it seems we have had a skeleton in our own closet all along, and it hardly makes sense to react by cursing the man who uncovered the evidence that it is there. Rather it is time for objective determination of answers to some of the many questions which come to mind. How many people are adversely affected by the *Solanaceae*? What health problems other than arthritis are involved? What alkaloids are involved in the Solonaceae; which one or ones are likely the most potentially dangerous? Are they genetically linked? What levels of which alkaloids do we have in *Solanaceae* cultivars? What can horticultural science *do* about this? And, as Norman Childers himself has been saying all along, we need research in human nutrition and medical science as well to get some of the needed answers.

This is a challenge to horticultural science, not a threat. And it can be neither ignored nor swept under the rug. Enormous industries are involved in the *Solonaceae.* Objective research is needed to define the extent of the difficulty, the population involved, and potential solutions determined. Horticultural crops are suspect, and we are the science society for these crops. Clearly the leadership in this matter must come from the American Society for Horticultural Science. The challenge is there, and the need is now.

No matter what happens, there is a growing number like myself who will lead a normal life — without the *Solanaceae.* We are grateful to Norman Childers for that.

Arthur H. Thompson
University of Maryland

"OH MY ACHING BACK!"

Note: The following letter came from the same horticultural colleague at the Maryland Agricultural Experiment Station. He has probably trained more PhDs and Masters students in horticulture than any other living Horticultural professor in the USA. His research and teaching have been outstanding. NFC.

"I have just received the announcement of *the book,* and am responding with a check. I look forward to it, and have advertised it around here. My secretary told me today she is going to buy a copy for a friend.

"You are off to the Orient and won't see this for a month. But while I am at the typewriter I may as well "report in", as it were. For you don't know what happened to me.

"I turned 59 last month (1977). In reviewing my experiences, I can point the finger at an incident 17 yrs. ago which suggests my problems were beginning then. I bought a 1960 Pontiac wagon to pull my first trailer traveller. I didn't like the new models — the seats were too low which gave me trouble on long drives. My dealer raised the front seat of that Pontiac ½ inch, the maximum he could go. It helped, but I still didn't like it. I took a 3-month travel sabbatic in that rig in 1961; the seat was still too low, but the problem was moderate.

"Real troubles began when our motor pools bought new 1970 Ford sedans in the fall of 1969. When I got to the University Substation with one of those cars, I spent a few moments leaning on the hood to get my back straightened out before I walked to the lab bldg. It was serious enough to ask for GM and Chrysler cars after a few trips in those Fords. But I was getting worse. The 1970 Ford experience told me I had a real problem; it was all downhill after that. My coworker has done the stoop jobs since 1971 while I have done the standup jobs, in measuring trunks, e.g. I bought a new Chevy in 1971 — a Chevy Blazer. This short wheelbase truck has chair-height seats; by this time I hated passenger cars because my back hurt so much. Getting out of bed in the morning was work.

"A thorough medical exam revealed no disc problem whatever. I was told I had "a little arthritis in the lower spine; nothing could be done about it. Take aspirin when the pain gets bad".

"1976 was my worst year. Daily living was a chore. I told my wife last winter she now is the family gardener by default — I simply could not bend over anymore. My one respite was walking, and I do much of that. But I was in such shape I was contemplating early retirement, moving to Wenatchee, Washington now rather than wait another few years. Perhaps the dry climate would help. I was getting to the end of my road."

"Pure chance put me in the same seat section with you on the flight to Cleveland last March. The bag of peanuts (Paprika labeled on the bag) offered by the stewardess changed my whole life, for that brought up the subject. I began avoiding the nightshades immediately, perhaps somewhat out of desperation, but also with the attitude of having nothing really whatever to lose, and a great deal to gain. I don't think I really believed it would do anything for my back, but I was most anxious to try.

"I responded before March was out. I woke up one morning vaguely aware that I had not awakened to turn my body over with the long familiar routine of manipulation of the elbows to minimize the pain in the back. A night or two later it happened again. Sure enough I had gone to sleep on one side, awakened on the other side! That had not happened in more than three years.

"That gets attention! Now I observed closely, but kept the business low key all the way. By early April, I was sleeping through the night without waking up to turn myself over. But I still had pain turning over *before* I went to sleep. So really it was no big deal. However, it turned out to be the beginning of a steady progression to a normal life. Painless sleep, easier driving of motor pool cars, a bit of weeding this spring and summer without problems then or later. Then on June 13th I arrived. I got out of bed that morning and strode to the picture window of our bedroom to view all my backyard plants — a routine of 21 years since we moved into that bedroom. But *this* morning I had gotten out of bed and strode to the window like any normal person! For the first time I had gotten up and walked away without standing still to get straightened up, or simply wait for that first back pain of the day. It *always* began then. And so for me June 13th was the day.

"Two days later we left for a month on the road with our travel trailer — Nashville, Dayton, Purdue (peach pruning), Rochester, Duluth, Thunder Bay, Ottawa, Ithaca, New York. Several times I got caught as a guest with the nightshades before me. I first got by as best I could, but by the time I got to Cornell in Ithaca, I decided it was time to put it all to test anyhow. When the Mrs. served a large bowl of wonderful potato salad, I made the most of it for I like the stuff. My departure from the Diet had been limited, and yet the last two mornings on the road I had the old back pains when I got out of bed in the trailer. Mild to be sure, but they were unmistakable.

"So now I am back on a tight schedule. Clearly, I am one who was going to hell fast with the *Solanaceae* and didn't know it. Now I am enjoying little things which I thought I had given up forever. An evening after dinner weeding ivy, holly, the garden with no ill effects. Perhaps even more significant — my professional life goes on to normal terms. I can look forward to finishing out my years here, then go back to Wenatchee to enjoy the climate rather than having the outlook of hoping that climate will correct something.

"And so it is with one case history. I have nothing but encouragement for your book. I have seen the bias of vegetable breeders when I tell 'em about my reaction to the nightshades, but I don't take any stuff from any of them. I tell 'em as researchers they ought to know better than scoff at evidence. But feelings run strong on this issue, and I can well imagine some of the flak that will follow your book. But it is as I tell my wife and my graduate students, my lifelong motto of sorts holds that, "The truth makes you free". And so I lean on that when contemplating the reception of your book. Best wishes in this endeavor." AHT:MD.

NIGHTSHADES — WE'RE STILL IN THE DARK!

The Arthritis Foundation of Westfield, N. J. 25 Prospect St., 07090, issued the following statement to their subscribers in May 1980.

A book titled "The Nightshades and Health" has recently received some publicity, though it was published more than two years ago. Principal author and publisher is Norman F. Childers, a professor of Horticulture at Rutgers — the State University of New Jersey. He makes the claim that four foods — tomatoes, white potatoes, garden peppers and eggplant (plus tobacco) — are toxic and cause arthritis, and their elimination from the diet controls the disease. He does not claim cure.

A long list of other problems in addition to arthritis have been corrected by the diet, he says, such as tender nipples in men, sluggish mind, and lack of ambition. He used "cooperators" to try his diet and report back, resulting in a collection of favorable case histories. The research and "survey" evidence cited in support of the claims does not offer reliable proof of a connection between diet and arthritis.

It seems difficult for the Foundation to accept diet as a cause of arthritis, even though the medical profession has rejected a bacteria, a fungus, or possibly a virus as the cause. They do not know the cause, but they do claim that gout is caused by diet, which is contradictory. NFC.

ADVICE GIVEN BY MODERN MATURITY MAGAZINE

Diets Won't Reduce Arthritic Pain! By Valerie Kelly

QUESTION: *I have painful bouts of osteoarthritis in my joints. A friend who is also afflicted tells me she has kept hers under control for some time by changes she's made in her diet.*

She drinks a certain kind of tea and has stopped eating some foods such as tomatoes and potatoes.

I'm wondering if I should try her prescription.

ANSWER: The only prescriptions you should use are those dispensed by your physician and you'd do well to take your friend's diet with the proverbial grain of salt.

The **Arthritis Foundation** advises people with this common form of arthritis to forget about special diets. There is no scientific evidence that eating or foregoing specific foods has any value whatever in treating or "curing" osteoarthritis.

You should eat a normal, well-balanced diet of varied, nourishing foods. If you're overweight, however, you may need a reducing diet to lessen the stress on weight-bearing joints.

Aches and pains and stiffness of arthritis flare up and then may lessen or subside on their own for periods of time. Persons who happen to be trying food fads and other gimmicks may attribute the temporary improvement to these essentially worthless remedies.

Osteoarthritis, like other forms of arthritis, is a chronic disease. However, a good, long-range treatment program under medical supervision can ease pain, maintain joint mobility, prevent disability, slow down and control the disease.

So seeing your doctor and following his orders makes far more sense than taking a friend's advice, no matter how well-intentioned it is.

For an informative, free booklet, "Arthritis: The Basic Facts," contact your local chapter of the Arthritis Foundation. If you're unable to locate a chapter in your area, write to: Arthritis Foundation, Lenox Post Office Box 18888, Atlanta, Ga. 30326. Enclose a self-addressed, stamped envelope.

LETTERS TO MODERN MATURITY MAGAZINE

Dear Editor:

I was very disappointed to read in "What Should I Do?" column, Sept. 1979, the answer to the arthritis question.

I have had osteoarthritis for five years and have not been without pain. I had changed my lifestyle to "easing around" to avoid aggravating my condition. Two months ago I started a Diet which eliminated foods of the nightshade family and I have been free of arthritic pain since then. I have gone from taking anti-flammatory drugs and 15 aspirin per day (on my doctors recommendation) to 4 aspirin per day. I have also been able to resume normal physical activity without pain. My hands aren't stiff every morning anymore. My whole life has been changed because of this Diet and your article calls it a "worthless remedy" and "no value whatever". *I am appalled!*

Would it have been wrong to suggest to the person who was inquiring that it certainly wouldn't hurt to cut these four foods out of their diet on a trial basis? You could still have a "well-balanced diet of varied nourishing foods" without using the nightshades. You could still follow your doctor's orders while trying this diet. I did.

If you knew of this diet, developed by Dr. Norman F. Childers, and still answered as you did, SHAME ON YOU. If you were unaware of his work (he has records to prove that 1000s of people have been helped by this Diet) I suggest you write to him. JHR:Ala. *(Note: No interest indicated. NFC)*

I WAS SO ANGRY

Note: The following letter was sent to the Arthritis Foundation in Atlanta, Georgia. I was so angry when I read "your" article, or the person representing you, on page 43 of the August-September 1979 MODERN MATERITY Magazine. Until December 18, 1978, I would have accepted all your conclusions. On that important date of my life I was fortunate to read about Dr. Norman F. Childers' "No-Nightshades Diet". Having suffered with painful arthritis for 25 years, I was feeling worse every year. I have been on this Diet for 10 months, and feel better and better as times goes by. You will never convince me that omitting the nightshades from my diet has not accomplished this.

Since you are supported by public funds and donations I believe that you must start to give publicity in some manner for sufferers to try this Diet. What have they got to lose but pain? What will you lose? Nothing, but gratitude from a suffering public!

Remember Sister Kenny and the abuse she suffered from organized medicine. Do take this program to heart, and try to find out why the nightshades have been causing these problems to us victims. I do hope to see a constructive attitude from the Arthritis Foundation. FG:N.Y.

BLOOD PRESSURE NOW NORMAL

I have read your book and adhere strictly to the Diet. My arthritis is not really severe, but at times it can be discomforting. I'm thinking in preventative terms. I am feeling much better and while I have high blood pressure and am taking medication, my blood pressure at this writing is normal. I attribute this to your Diet. BFM:Pa.

BEST MONEY I EVER SPENT ON MYSELF

I am 72 and have had health problems since I started walking at 11 mos of age. I cried they said when picked up. The doctors said hurts in knees, hips and shoulders were only "growing pains". At 12 mos I never walked again until I was five yrs when I was placed in a walker that my brother pushed around forcing me to start walking. In the early 1950s I came down with rheumatoid arthritis and became completely helpless. Doctors gave me gold shots and cortisone and I finally recovered. The doctor told me it was up to me to walk and I fought hard and won. About 4 yrs ago I had arthritis of the spine, with pain down the side of the left leg. It was excruciating. Doctor wanted to operate but I declined with a flat "No!" One day about 2 yrs ago I saw an article about your work and at the end it said there was a book to buy and I thought they were looking for another sucker to buy a book. But I could not seem to put the idea of those vegetables out of my mind and finally wrote for the book. It was the best $20 I ever spent on myself. I figured I had tried about everything and had nothing to lose but pain. I was eating potatoes and tomatoes as if they were going out of style, always had, plus peppers, pizza and eggplant off and on. After several mos. on the Diet, I noticed that on awakening in the morning I could for the first time close my hand into a fist. I also could get right out of bed and walk without staggering against the wall. What a wonderful relief. I do not recall a day in my life until a few months ago that I did not have at least fleeting pains in some joint in my body. Also, I used to have facial neuralgia, headaches and earaches. When the weather is bad I still can feel some small pains, or when I get a cold, but they are nothing like they used to be. Maybe I shall never get rid of all pains but thank God most of them are gone. MGB:Ky.

WE SLEEP GOOD NIGHTS NOW!

We received the Newscard you circulated to cooperators telling us about all the things to avoid. Both my wife and I have been feeling real good as far as aches and pains are concerned. We have been staying free from eating any of the nightshades for well over a year now. We watch what we buy very carefully to be sure we do not get paprika and the like in bought foods. We sleep good almost every night because of being free from pains that used to wake us. My wife's knees used to swell quite often but she is never bothered any more. We appreciate hearing from you in the Newscards and any new ideas to keep ourselves well. Sorry we have not answered sooner.

I wish more people I know would become interested in the problem with the nightshade plants and foods. But most people like to eat everything they have eaten all their lives — tomatoes, potatoes, peppers, etc. Thanks to you, we became wise and are living real good and happily now. CEL:N.Y.

SOME ITALIANS CAN DO THE DIET!

I have been taking bufferin and the like for years. They have helped somewhat. But I have been in almost constant pain for all of 18 yrs. At times it has become unbearable to walk around crippled and with a stiff neck. I have tried to get help for yrs. from doctors but to no avail. They all just say — "arthritis." About once a week I would get a severe attack when my ankles, wrists and neck would swell and really become painful. And about 4-5 days later the swelling would go down with no apparent permanent effect. I would tell this to the doctors and at times, show them — but the answer was always, "arthritis"! So many times I would suggest to them that it might be the lack of something in my system, or, in fact, too much of some substance. I went through this over and over again for years and always without help from M.D.s.

Accidentally, I read a note in Prevention magazine about your research and I immediately sent for the book. It was a "God send." I immediately eliminated the nightshades and got relief within a week or so.I still have some aches but nothing like the pains of the past. Now, I can walk like a normal human being.

Dr. Childers, I wish to point out to you that my being an Italian makes it hard to follow your Diet 100%. In Italian foods a lot of tomatoes, peppers, potatoes and eggplants are used. I am a businessman and have to eat out a lot so it makes it doubly difficult but I do watch carefully and will continue to do so.

My big question is whether researchers or someone can take these toxins out of the nightshades, process them out or breed them out, so we Italians can continue to eat the nightshades. In conclusion, I can only say that I am forever grateful to you and your cooperators for the research you have done. SB:Fla.

Note: This man is 60 yrs., 175 lbs., had a heart fibrillation, some skin cancer, and benign tumors and moles, which often go with heavy nightshades consumption.

GINGER ROOT SEASONING?

I am still improving. No pains but I still have a problem getting through the night sometimes. You pointed out that lomitil pills have atropine (nightshade) in them so I quit taking them. I have a real problem with ginger root seasoning. Within 20 minutes after eating it, I have pains. Field peas and beets also affect me. My husband went on this diet and also stopped smoking. His hips have stopped hurting and he tells everybody about the nightshades. Some think he is nuts. His sister is an R.N. and she hoots at him but she also has arthritis. She has a tomato plant 6 ft. tall that bears buckets of tomatoes. I am so grateful we found out about the Diet. RLS:Tx.

HIKING 400 + MILES, 67 YRS OLD, WAS VERY ARTHRITIC!

Note: This man started the Diet in November 2⅔ yrs before his final report. Presented here are his initial casing of his situation and progress reports. His case is well documented and reason for presenting it in full. NFC.

I am 64 yrs, 125 lbs, had my problems for 5 and 18 yrs, knees, shoulders and back are bothersome, have been eating as many as 21 lbs of potatoes a week and relatively little of the other nightshades and I do not smoke. I have some digestive discomfort at times, no skin rashes, no heart problem or cancer but do have pre-cancers on the face, and an assortment of moles on my back and many liverspots. My right knee muscles tire easily for I have been jogging 2-5x/wk since my teens. I had osteomyelitis just above the joint when 12 yrs of age. My left knee has osteoarthritis since 1960, or 18 yrs. X-rays showed calcium accumulation and ordinary walking okey but I cannot jog consecutive days. My back by X-rays shows spurs since 1960s, also cause of abdominal and groin surface sensations. Back pain was partially relieved with heel lift, 1970. Both shoulders are bothered, "frozen shoulders," restricted movement, soreness which was partially relieved by Dong/Banks Diet. My digestive track discomfort has been helped some by high fiber diet. I am a regular listener of Dr. Carleton Fredericks' program on WOR, New York, and he told about your work in November when I went on this Diet with the descriptions above. Following is my progress.

As of 6 months after starting the Childers' Diet, it is working! There is no doubt in my mind that the nightshades are the culprit — possibly the only one.

Report Intervals and Methods: In my case, much as you predicted, improvement is slow. Hence, the intervals between reports is long. At the time I entered your cooperative test I had been on the Diet for over two months. I kept a diary and criteria. The diary I keep is in the form of a chart with approximately 12 entries for each date. Up-date is made about twice a month. Criteria are both subjective and objective. Objective criteria, preferable, of course, has been difficult for me to formulate and as you will see applicable only in the case of my shoulders.

Right and Left Shoulders: Slowly, my "frozen shoulders," a condition dating back to 1973, are thawing:

Subjective criteria:

1. Shoulders permit sleeping on back only.
2. Shoulders permit sleeping on right or left side after initial period of sleep.
3. Shoulders permit sleeping on one side only, initially.
4. Shoulders permit sleeping on either side, initially.
5. No shoulder pain detectable in bed regardless of position or movement.

Since November at the start, I have progressed from about 2 plus to about 4 plus on the subjective scale.

Objective Criteria:

1. Distance fingers of one hand can be made to extend over and back of opposite shoulder.
2. Height arm behind back can be raised relative to opposite hip.
3. Height to which hands can be extended above head.

While all three showed progress in joint mobility, #2 and #3 were most sensitive to joint condition. Criterion #3, in particular, showed a consistent and marked improvement. A further subjective indication of improvement is the fact that I can now do push-up exercises — something I have not been able to do for 5 yrs.

Back:

Subjective indications only.

Since starting to use a heel lift in 1970, I have not been bothered by the usual variety of back pain caused by muscle spasm induced by "pinched nerves". Recent manifestations have been in the form of tight and/or burning abdominal sensations; also surface sensations of the abdominal and groin areas. I was told by a doctor that the groin area discomfort originated from arthritis of the coccyx. The spinal and coccyx arthritis induced pains have not been chronic. Recently, they have been experienced 4 or 5 times a year and are triggered by either of two identified activities: certain stretching movements or sitting-up exercises. I have not had a recurrence for approximately 6 months. I also have observed that the stretching movements that in the past caused an attack, no longer do so. I am also finding that I can take sitting-up exercises without triggering an attack.

Left Knee:

Subjective criteria, only. These are:

1. Pain when crawling or kneeling on knee.
2. Pain in walking or running up stairs.
3. Pain in jogging; frequency of jogging permitted.
4. Pain in running.

The first three criteria activities have been indulged in both before and after going on the Childers' Diet. They all gave trouble before but now are nearly trouble-free. My knee is no longer the limiting factor in jogging. I can jog consecutive days, the distance being limited by endurance, not by knee. For the first time in years I can run short distances without pain.

Additional Remarks:

While I have made a lot of progress, I have a considerable distance to go. Shoulder/arm mobility can be considerably improved. I still get occasional indication from knee and back that not all is completely well. Twice, I have had general set-backs. Both were when I had a cold or virus, which I hold responsible. For the past two years I have been on a mega-vitamin/full spectrum mineral (except copper) regimen. Aside from arthritis, I have felt better on this regimen. At your suggestion I did reduce the vitamin D intake. Obviously, I have no indication whether the regimen has helped or hindered the arthritis program. A long-term ambition has been that of hiking the length of the Appalachian Trail when I retire. If I succeed completely or in part, you will have been the person who made it possible.

Twenty-two months after starting the Diet, we find that this cooperator is still rigidly on the Diet, taking thyroid pills, vitamins, not smoking, and says, "Back and knee continue to improve — *knee improvement is amazing*. Currently jogging 4-6 miles/day and walking another 2-3 miles. Shoulders are on a plateau with little change the past 12 months"

Thirty-one months after starting the Diet, he says, "You may be interested that I, a former arthritic, am successively hiking the Appalachian Trail, retired, starting in Georgia September 27 last, and now in Damascus, Virginia, a distance of 446 miles. The Childers' No-Nightshades Diet has made this possible. Feeling fine! More later when I arrive in New Jersey. GLG:N.J.

Note: We have been watching a number of arthritics in this immediate area and have noted that age does not seem to make much difference when they start the Diet and while badly disfigured people will show gradual improvement, obviously so, those who are not so badly affected also will show very gradual improvement as long as we have had opportunity to watch and that has been close to 6 years. So we wish to be encouraging to you who may be in this condition at the start. Stay with the Diet as rigidly as you possibly can and you should be rewarded as the months pass. This is really the first definite hope, I believe, in history that anyone could offer you. Arthritics are discarding canes, walkers and wheelchairs. N.F.C.

INDULGENCE NOT WORTH WEEK-LONG "HANGOVER"!

I am 57 yrs and have had the problem only about a year before a student in my Tai Chi class told me about your article in Prevention magazine. I eliminated all but the potato which she did not mention, so when your book arrived I stopped that and a few months later am now free of all pain — mainly my hip. Last July 4 I indulged in baked beans that are in a tomato sauce mix. For the following four days my leg ached so badly I went back on aspirin for relief. Now I am free of pain again. I have had to give up all those previous foods that I really like but indulgence is simply not worth the week-long hangover. My sister has stopped the nightshades too and now she can snap her fingers for the first time in three years. I have flare-ups after eating spinach, beets and asparagus. Thank you for the nightshades information — I kiss your hand, Dr. Childers! DC:Ca.

ARTHRITIS SETTLED IN KNEE INJURY AT 19 YRS

I am 67 yrs, 210 lbs, 6' 2'', and have had bad arthritic problems in feet, ankles, shoulders, neck and particularly in my knee. After a yr on the Diet, all aches and pains have disappeared. Overwork, however, will bring tired aching feet and ankles, which I assume is normal. My results have been so good that I intend to continue the Diet. While my arthritic problems generally have been bad for 12 yrs, my knee damaged in soccer has bothered me since 19 yrs of age. I was a constant smoker (which I stopped last year) and loved tomatoes. WD:Canada.

PSORIASIS AND CHOCOLATE

I had psoriasis on my elbows and knees since childhood and learned late in life that chocolate caused it. To this day if I eat chocolate (2 Hershey bars), I will develop a spot the size of a quarter on my knees; a quantity will cause my finger joints to ache with little bumps forming there. I was addicted to chocolate and do not keep it in the house. CN:IDA

TWITCHS IN HANDS CORRECTED

I abstained from all nightshades but occasionally had a baked potato that was the culprit causing twitches in my hands. Stupid — I just could not imagine an innocent, white, easy-to-digest potato doing that. It was a lucky day when I hobbled to your meeting in Somerville, N. J. over four years ago. I have been without pain now for the full time. Please change my address to Pennsylvania. HEW:Pa.

HAD ARTHRITIS SINCE 13 YRS

I have suffered with arthritis since I was 13 yrs of age and I am now 26. I have undergone X-rays and blood tests but the doctor says I do not have rheumatoid arthritis but some other kind. After hearing about your Diet, I figured it would not hurt to stop the vegetables you mentioned. The difference I have felt is remarkable. Can you send me more information? DS:N.J.

ONE SPLURGE LASTED A WEEK

''While in Florida on vacation, I won two dinners at a ''Taco'' restaurant and was going to forget it, but my wife said why not go to see if my ''allergy'' had left. So, I told the waitress to go light on any hot stuff. Well, the next day I could hardly get in and out of my trailer. That food really hit me and it lasted for several days. Within a week I was about 90% which is back to almost normal for me. My knees still had some soreness and ache. I no longer have any back problems, however, my friends think I am crazy for NOT eating the nightshades.'' G.E.H.:NJ

Note: This man was 67 when he started the Diet 4 years earlier. He hurt his back 30 years previously lifting baled hay.

SWOLLEN FROZEN JOINTS

I put off writing, thinking I'd get some snapshots made of my joints and trying to find pictures of me when I was so bad — but I just don't have any that really show — since I wasn't too keen on having my picture taken then! I wish too, that I had taken measurements of my fingers, ankles and knees to show the extent of swelling I had and how little I have now.

I think that finally I am "clean" of the nightshades. For two months now, I know I have not eaten anything that contained the tiniest bit of pepper or potato starch (they were hidden culprits for me). I don't trust many prepared or bought foods, do most of my cooking from scratch and just don't eat if I am in a place where there is doubt about the foods! I also have not taken any vitamin pills for these last two months (that was hard for me because I was a firm believer in vitamin C and E).

I ordered your book August 7, 1978 so I have been eliminating nightshades from my diet since 1st of September 1978. I am suspicious of all foods now where, at first, I would eat things never realizing they had hidden ingredients (took me a long time before I found out some candies have potato starch in them). I do not eat many sweets any more and substitute fruits instead.

I see progress every day in the use of my joints. My knees are frozen in a sitting position so I cannot stand up, but I practice kicking my legs out and find I go a little farther each day. The knees are beginning to have movement in the joints and *without pain* which is miraculous to me. I am able to do exercises with my atrophied muscles in my legs so I am getting some strength again. I do every exercise slowly and deliberately and firmly believe that I will use my legs again.

My wrists were also frozen but I can bend them some. Exercise with them and my hands is *not painful.*

The best thing yet though is my frame of mind. I do not have that terrible depression since I got rid of nightshades. I took my last Nalfon pill September 8, 1978 and have not had an aspirin, etc., in months. Thank you again and again for the work you are doing. Mrs. JSW: Ky., USA

Note: This lady in 1978 was 55 yrs., had the problem for 7 yrs., did not smoke, weight 146 lbs., ate potatoes 3-4x/wk., peppers daily, eggplant occasionally, paprika daily, pizza 1/wk., no other severe health problems, except occasional dizziness, headaches, ear problems and pleurisy.

DIETED SKEPTICALLY

"I am over 40 years and diagnosed with arthritis in the hip which has been giving me problems the past year. I saw an item on your theory, was beginning to think I had to give up my jogging, physical exercise, and as a last resort, skeptically, decided to try eliminating the nightshades from my diet. Only a month ago I stopped eating these foods and within days I noticed an improvement. It is rare now that I feel even a twinge of pain. I plan to continue the test for six months. Let me know if you need another cooperator." M.M.: Wa.

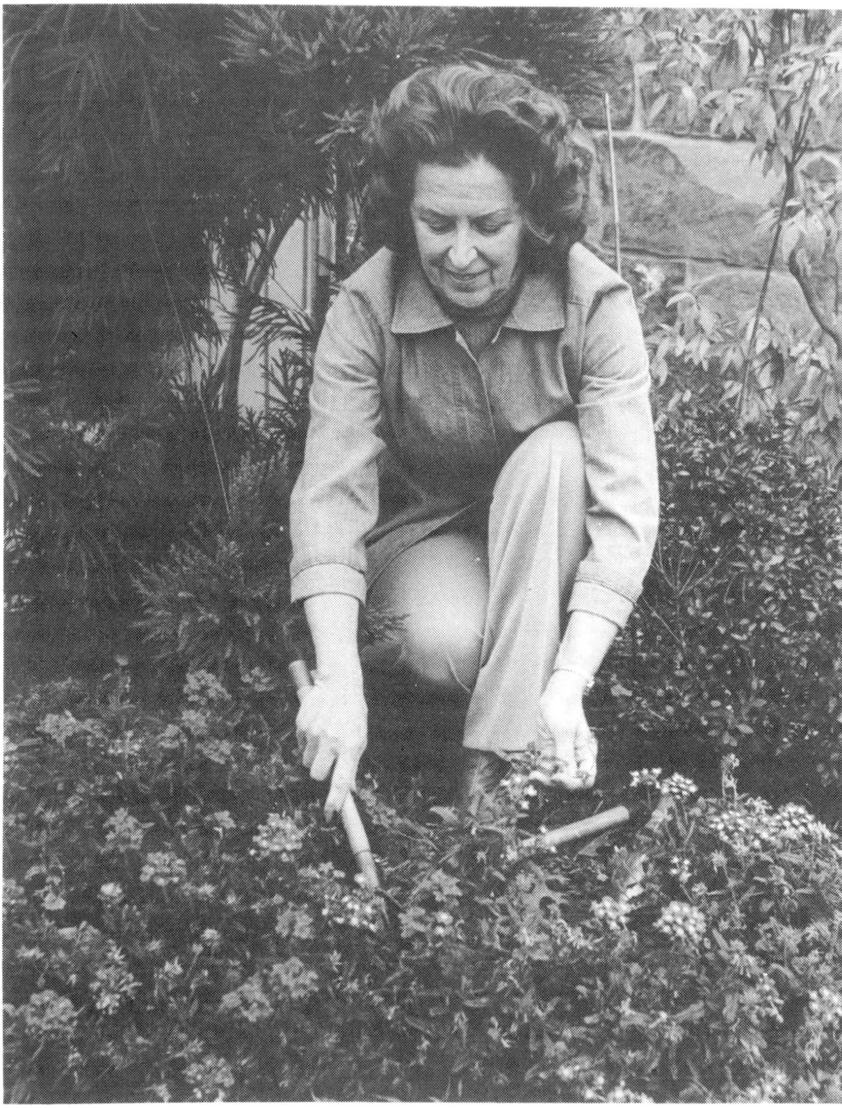

Mrs. Emily Osterman of New Jersey (above) writes, "I can now garden, keep house, do most anything with no problem. I want to tell you, Dr. Childers, how happy I am with your Diet which has been followed rigidly for over 4 yrs. I shall never go back to *those* foods again. Only a tiny bit of paprika will bring pains to my hips (X-rayed arthritic) and back and swelling in my hands. Whenever the old symptoms appear, I can always trace them back to a nightshade gotten unknowingly. I spread the word daily. Hundreds of people in this area are eternally grateful for your research and you. (Photo by Dick Costello, New Brunswick Home News).

CRIPPLED, IRRATIC LIFE SINCE 10.

It was an absolutely and completely satisfying pleasure to meet with you yesterday. I cannot express the happiness I feel today — I feel free at last! Free of the life-long fear that I would eat a food that would unknowingly result in a often repeated bed-ridden agony.

As I told you, I have severe diagnosed arthritis of the hips, knees, neck and wrists from which I have suffered since childhood. I first became aware of the severity at about age 10. I had swelling of the knees and could not play as others did. On and off through grammar school I visited the doctors, wore knee braces and had my knees drained by hypodermic needles, took cortisone (sometimes caused big purple blotches on my skin), aspirin and a number of recommended pain-killers. During high school I endured days in bed in severe pain, spent weeks on crutches, used the school freight elevator to get up and down floors. I was unable to walk stairs. During college at Lehigh I endured the same to a somewhat lesser degree since I had inadvertently begun to avoid some foods. One doctor had suggested losing weight (no potatoes) would help. I went from 180 to 155 lbs during early college.

Upon graduation and several years after, I noticed that foods and "weight" had an effect and I kept my weight down, but about once in every two weeks I'd have severe pain, swelling, sleeplessness, etc. During my 20s it grew much worse. The disability affected my job (I could not get over the floor well), my marriage (wife cooked Italian food), etc. I'm now divorced. I consulted many doctors, spent thousands of dollars, went month after month. Two surgeons wanted to operate. Fortunately, I found a doctor who suggested food allergy which aggravated the arthritis. Working with him I found a number of foods that did aggravate my aches and pains and swelling. About this time I was in bed much of the time and actually wished I were dead while filled with 10-20 aspirins a day. Without exaggeration, my problem was growing into a life-or-death struggle of work-family-health problems. I quickly found success and was back on my feet after avoiding a number of foods that included tomatoes and peppers, but I was still using potatoes in the diet. Occasionally, I did have bedridden problems but at least I could survive. I began to eat a steady diet of: Breakfast: Orange juice, muffin and black coffee; Lunch: Turkey, lettuce and cheese on white bread; and dinner: Fish, light vegetables and potato. If I kept strictly on this diet, I was "OK," but with mild pain much of the time. Any major "normal" food variation would cause problems. Over the past 10 yrs I have refined the diet by pinpointing problems and avoiding the following foods at any cost!

Tomato or tomato products of any kind
Spices of any kind
Nuts or seeds of any kind (may have had paprika on them)
Eggs (allergy or possibly had paprika on them) caused sore jaw

Red meats and gravies (meat sauce may have had spices, or, potato in the gravies to give it body)
Peas (Processed may have green berries from nightshade weed growing among peas)
Asparagus
Onions

It is with gratitude to you, that I now add *potato*. Undoubtedly, it was the unidentified fouling object. Note: I never eat eggplant, disliked it. I have read your book (in 5 straight hours). I absolutely support you with every swollen part of my body *(He apparently got a nightshade travelling and eating out a few days ago).* It all ties in. *You are right on!*

I have the desire to assist you and your efforts in any way I can. I know the pain and agony of the severely affected people. I have lived with it for 30 yrs. It has nearly ruined my life several times. It always made my life much less enjoyable. I want to help you spread the nightshades story. I gave the two extra books I bought to my relatives who also suffer severely. EW,Sr:N.J.

QUESTIONS?

"My husband and I suspect that solanine, or one of the chemicals in the nightshades, could be responsible for *deforming our two sons,* one of whom died. My husband is a veterinarian and I am a registered nurse. We know that more deformed babies are born in Ireland than any other country — due to Spina bifida (open spine), anencephaly (absence of brain cortex), and hydrocephaly (water head). Evidence indicates that this situation may be due to four factors in Ireland vs. Eastern Europe where twice as many potatoes per capita are eaten. (1) High humidity — 30 to 100 inches, rains 2 out of every 3 days; (2) diet is chiefly potatoes; (3) potatoes are stored raw, not dried into flour as in Eastern Europe, and, (4) potatoes are cooked and eaten with the peel (high in solanine). Major deformities in Boston have been shown to be 6 times more prevalent among Irish babies than among Jewish babies, latter of whom eat less potatoes. This has been determined not to be due to a genetic weakness. We know that potato stems, leaves and sprouts are poisonous to people and livestock. Solanine is not destroyed by cooking. Potatoes must be stored properly (away from light) or solanine will increase markedly in the tubers. We have much more evidence I have searched out and will be glad to correspond if interested." N.H.:Wis.

THE REAL McCOY!

"We read the article about your work with arthritis in the Philadelphia Evening Bulletin over 6 months ago and started the Diet immediately. My wife and I are both very grateful to you. Dr. Childers, you are not a faith healer but The Real McCoy. Our aches, pains, fluid-on-the-knees have completely disappeared." B.R.:Pa.

WAS IN A WHEELCHAIR — NOW PHYSICALLY ACTIVE.

I have suffered from arthritis for about 10 years, am 66, a farmer. The attacks became progressively more painful and disabling. Pain would be felt around the joints but not within them. The thighs would be affected after sitting for some time. Areas around some joints (ankles, knees, fingers, wrists) would become swollen and painful to the touch. I was medically diagnosed on 2 occasions as having a "gouty" situation resulting from excessive uric acid. I was placed on a diet to reduce uric acid, but no restrictions on the nightshades. Some improvement was noted. A second diagnosis of a uric acid problem was noted later with a test level of 8.2 (normal range of 4 to 8). Daily dosage of 200 mg of Zyloprim (Allopurinol) was prescribed which helped some but attacks continued.

Last summer while on Zyloprim I experienced my worst attack and became a candidate for 3-wheel all-terrain cycle chair which enabled me to perform my livestock duties. My left knee and hip and right ankle had excruciating pain simultaneously. After reading an item in Organic Gardening, "A diet to Stop Arthritis", I eliminated the nightshades from my diet. At that time I was consuming tomatoes several times a day, baked potatoes daily and ingesting their jackets as well. Japanese eggplant and peppers were consumed occasionally from my garden. After eliminating the nightshades I could see a difference in 3 days and after 1½ wks I was almost back to normal. However, pain in shoulders persisted after a night's sleep and was the last to disappear. In the meantime I ordered your book, "The Nightshades and Health."

At this time after about 6 months, I am virtually painfree and more physically active than I have been in 10 yrs. I have not taken any medication (Zyloprim) for about 2 months. I feel great! I am eternally grateful for your findings and so very thankful that I chanced to read the article about your Diet. The quality of my life and outlook for the future are tremendously improved. Thank you, thank you. REH:Ca..

MY CRIPPLED FRIENDS — STUBBORN, WON'T BELIEVE, WON'T SACRIFICE

I am 69 yrs, had neck, back, shoulder and hip problems and was eating a nightshade(s) daily. Results have been fabulous. Three yrs after starting the Diet, we moved so that interfered with my Diet and I have had some aches and pains again. When I follow the diet and watch out for all the nightshades, I feel fine. Paprika is my biggest enemy because it is so hidden. Dr. Childers, when I see some of my friends and how they are crippled and suffering with arthritis, I thank God for you and all you have done for us. I find them stubborn, won't believe or just don't want to make any sacrifices. VMB:N.J.

CONFUSED — BUT FEEL GREAT!

I was a tomato and potato hound. I am 57, weight 130 lbs and have had arthritis for 3 yrs. Doctor advised 6 aspirins a day but they only mask the problem while it gets worse, so I was doing without aspirin and tolerating the pain. I have had no pain since a few days after I stopped eating the nightshades. Before this, however, I had been to a chiropractor who checked my allergies and said I was allergic to a lot of foods but *not* peppers and tomatoes. He also said I was allergic to metamucil which I was taking for diverticulosis. With a hair analysis he said I was deficient in zinc, chromium, sodium and potassium but had excessive amounts of lead, mercury, cadmium (I thought only ghetto kids had excess lead from eating wallpaper and paint). At any rate I started on the detoxification program and your Diet at the same time and within a week I have felt great. So at this point I cannot tell you whether it is his program or your Diet. Incidentally, your book is being read avidly by all the neighbors with and without arthritic problems. JPI:Mass.

Note: She was advised by me to go off the Childers' Diet for two weeks and see what happens, or eat only peppers and tomatoes to which she is "not allergic", and see what happens. NFC.

WAS USING A CANE, NOW VERY ACTIVE, HEARING BETTER!

This is to inform you that I am one of your "cured" arthritics. Thanks to an announcement of your forthcoming book I am free of stiff joints and painful movement. During the last 8 yrs I was becoming more and more crippled in the knees, hip and feet. I am 47, a mother of 5, a housewife, returned to college for a degree in music. I was in a great deal of pain trying to play the pipe organ and walking up and down stairs. I hadn't played tennis for at least two years and was getting fat and lazy. Last March I could not walk without a cane, so I went to an orthopod who gave me cortisone shots and motrin. The motrin made me feel very tired all the time,so last June when your article appeared in the Providence Journal, I started your Diet and within three weeks I enjoyed much mobility and started to exercise again. Six months later I am more active than ever — hold down a job in medical malpractice claims dept. of an insurance company, teach music to 14 students in my studio, sing in the church choir twice a week, dance and act in several programs a year. My hearing is much improved. I am jogging with a dog 10 minutes every morning, losing weight and able to wear the clothes I like! My doctor was impressed, is telling other patients about it. Four days ago I tested tomatoes and hurt badly the following two days. These foods are poisonous to me. I want to thank you sincerely for your wonderful work. BJC:R.I.

QUIT ALL NIGHTSHADE FOODS AT ONCE, PLUS CIGARETTES

I had been toying with the idea of quitting cigarettes for some time when I saw an item about your Diet in my health store. It really hit home since I had been eating voraciously out of my garden and was getting sicker and sicker. Well, it has been about 6 wks now on the Diet and I am feeling much better, in fact, better than I have ever felt in my life. *(Another letter after 5 months follows)* I have felt so much better that I enrolled in a Tech. school machine shop training course. This spring I shall finish an Associate of Arts Degree in Education. It is not too much of an accomplishment but makes me feel real good. I can now see life differently. If anyone would have told me ten years ago that I would feel like this today, I would have laughed. I don't have the depression. I have much more stamina, and I certainly see life differently. I am grateful for your research. I don't know where I would have been today if I had not heard about this Diet. I may have been dead by now as I was very sick. Have a good Xmas and New Year. LF:Mo.

THE ANSWER TO THE ARTHRITIS PLAGUE

I am 59 yrs, 97 lbs., had problems for 10 yrs in hands, shoulders, neck and back, exercise only by walking, cannot dunk in ocean anymore. I have had osteopathic help for 19 yrs, am a vegetarian, but started your Diet last June. My finger joints were enlarged, stiff, but now I can move them around much more. I have had both shoulders dislocated several times and have to be extremely cautious in reaching, so I cannot participate in any sport. Now (subsequent letter) after 2 yrs+ on your Diet, I must say I believe your research and Diet will prove to be the answer to the arthritis plague. May you continue to be successful in all your endeavors. JM:N.Y.

SURGERY DEFERRED, MAYBE NOT NEEDED

I have been faithful on the Diet for 7 mos. I am aware of much less stiffness and distortion in fingers. My tenosynovitis in hands and wrists has diminished and surgery has been delayed; it may not be needed. On two occasions when I ate potatoes, I experienced strong pain and feverishness in index fingers, relived by aspirin. I am now confident that the Diet is slowly helping me. I am 72, 107 lbs, had problems over 10 yrs, taken all kinds of drugs, walk but have stopped swimming, and I learned to be left-handed due to bad right hand. I had a wrist brace and used hot water a lot. I have had osteoporosis, with nodes in many places, even in my jaw. I have had on occasion very bad bursitis, tennis elbow. I was not helpless but getting that way fast. Thank you for the Diet. LS:N.Y.

HIP OPERATION? NO! AN ASTONISHING RESULT!

I want to thank you for sending me your book,'' Nightshades and Health,'' as a gift from my good friend in North Plainfield, N.J. I have not written to you sooner because up to this time I have had very little to report. However, I took a great interest in the book, read it carefully, and tried to the best of my ability to find the foods to which I was allergic. After almost a year, I think that I can say with certainity that tomatoes and potatoes are the main offenders for me. After steadily eliminating them from my diet, I have seen an astonishing result.

The almost continuous pain that I have suffered the past five years is decreasing and I am able to walk much better. In fact, I frequently forget my cane and leave it somewhere.

I broke my hip in early 1970. I recovered with very little permanent injury (or so it seemed then) and I was able to look after my house, my garden and could walk for miles without tiring. Then I developed arthritis in my injured hip joint. Whenever there was pressure on my hip or I moved it, I suffered acute pain. I even walked with crutches at times. The doctor advised that I had a choice: (a) an operation, (b) drugs for pain, or (c) suffer. I chose to suffer. It was at this point that my friend came to visit me and then asked you to send your book. It was two weeks ago that I felt sure enough to write you. Again, thanks, and I shall keep you informed. EG:Md.

FRIENDS STUBBORN — WON'T TOLERATE DIET!

My pains are all gone! Some pains, as in my feet, that I had not attributed to arthritis I find are gone also. It certainly has been easy — with excellent results. I intend to continue this Diet for the rest of my life! I tell my friends about the Diet. They are stubborn and seemingly under no conditions would tolerate the Diet restrictions. MLM:N.J.

I AM A LABEL-READER

I saw an article in the Philadelphia Bulletin late 1978, checked the encyclopedia on nightshades and immediately went on the Diet. I am 70 yrs, have had arthritis and indigestion since I was 40. It came on slowly with arthritis of the neck, shoulders, hips and knees. Have taken aspirin, Bufferin, Anacin, Tylenol, Indocin, Clinoril, Naprosyn, you name it! A year and a half after starting the Diet, I am still on it rigidly. I am convinced that it is for me! Am on *no* medication and my stomach and arthritis rarely bother me anymore. I am off coffee, it seemed to upset me and I avoid spices and paprika completely. Chocolate bothers me. But, now I am about 99% free of aches and pains of any kind. I tell my friends but they do not believe me. ES:N.J.

GETTING OFF ALL PILLS IS GOOD

Continuing Diet and continue to improve. After eating several chocolates, I got a flareup the next day in my hands. I agree that getting off the pills if you are taking them ''just in hopes'', is a good idea. Bit by bit I am getting off them. Did you know that the Arthritis Foundation believes diet plays no part in arthritis? Ridiculous, I say. When I recognized a nightshade vine all over my yard with black berries, yellow bloom like a tomato *(Solanum dulcamura,* known as European bitter sweet), I cleared it out and got my aches and pains of arthritis back the next day. Can the toxins be absorbed by the skin *(answer is, Yes. The berries of this plant are poisonous if eaten in quantity. NFC).* ES:Ct.

CAUSED RED ITCHY EYES

I was on your Diet from February to August. My osteoarthritis of 8 years duration seemed to have lessened somewhat. In August, I intentionally broke the Diet with a dinner of white potatoes and tomatoes. The next morning my eyes were red and itchy, I felt toxic and my hands had needle like pains that had disappeared on the Diet. In addition, my knees and thoracic vertebrae were quite painful. After two days of eating potatoes, I was so uncomfortable that I went back on the Diet and have remained on it to date (9 mos. later).

In a few days I plan again to test myself off the Diet. I will report the results to you.

I have found it difficult to avoid pepper in public, and sometimes I think I get the needle like joint pains in my fingers, toes, and knees when I have eaten in a restaurant.

I also notice a marked improvement in a long standing allergic rhinitis (nose mucous membrane inflammation) after I started the Diet and it returned along with the red eyes when I broke the Diet last August.

Thanks for your interest. Has any of the arthritis centers shown any interest in your work? JRC-M.D.:Wash., D.C.

OFF MEDICINE, ON THE DIET

I heard Dr. Carleton Fredericks speak of your Diet on WOR, NYC, recently. I have been to many doctors prescribing all kinds of medicine. I have asked the doctors if diet played a part in arthritis and they all assured me, ''absolutely not''! I was just sure otherwise and when I heard Dr. Fredericks' program, I decided to quit the pills that made me dizzy and quit eating the foods mentioned as No, Nos. In only 2 wks my thumbs quit shooting pains, the third week I could sew, cut cloth, write and pick up jars without pain with much more strength. Then, gradually, I noticed my back was feeling so much better. I walked quicker and easier. Now I feel as I did 10 yrs ago. I am certainly going to stick with the Diet, but I am interested in knowing if you have published lists of where all the nightshades are found in food. Please write. FB:N.Y.

TOBACCO SMOKE INCREASES PAIN?

I have been on the No-Nightshades diet for over a year and swelling and pain has stopped in my fingers within two months after starting. I seem to have to take vitamin E because after one day without it I have cramps in my feet at night. *(Note: it was suggested she check this indicaton to be sure. We have a few cooperators who have a foot problem they seem not to be able to correct).* I have avoided sugar and tobacco smoke for years having found they cause increased pain. RCN:N.C.

EYES IMPROVED ON DIET!

Due to my diabetes my eyes were deteriorating, but when I had them checked after being on the Diet for about four months, the doctor said there were no more signs of deterioration, or any sign of eye disease. I do not know if the Diet was responsible for that *(Note: we have a few other cooperators who report this improvement. NFC)*

I find some small bakery goods in this area of Arkansas as rolls, bread and donuts have potato flour in them, apparently, but are not so-labelled. I get kick-backs from them. Found out the hard way. *(Note: Use of potato flour in bakery goods seems more prevalent in the midwest USA).* Thanks for all you have accomplished toward arthritic recoveries. I know — now I can write and knit! IB:Ark.

NIGHTSHADE BERRIES IN PEAS

I do not raise peas in my garden because I work in a cannery here in Washington and it is my job to pick the green nightshade berries out of the peas on the grading belt. The deadly nightshade *(Solanum nigrum)* is a weed in the pea fields and while most of the berries are black, the younger berries are green. We try to get them all out before canning. *(Note: This could explain why some cooperators have complained about canned and frozen peas giving them pains. The Washington Agricultural Experiment Station has a weed specialist on their staff to find chemicals to destroy the nightshade weed in pea fields but not harm the peas and, incidentally, this staff lady is one of our cooperators. NFC)* CMH:Wa.

PATIENTS RESPONDING!

We have gotten such good response with the first book that here is a check for another. This book has been very helpful with all my patients. Thank you so much for this fine research. Dr. KLL:N.C.; O.P.

PSORIASIS?

. . . . . I must add that my father used to have psoriasis and a friend told him that he also had psoriasis and that if my father would stop eating potatoes as he did, the problem would go away! KD:N.J.
Note: We have two cooperators who, too, have been freed of psoriasis with the diet.

ASK PROCESSORS TO OMIT NIGHTSHADES OR CLEARLY LABEL

"I was doing very well with the Diet until I fell on a slick pavement. Now I am recovering from hip damage. I am having trouble with *capsicum* (ground pepper) hidden in so many foods, potato too. I am also wondering if the chemicals in the nightshades can be absorbed through the skin *(answer is, yes).* I handle a lot of "Sevin" which is used to dust dogs for fleas and for garden pests. I find this and several other pesticides have a warning on the label that they are cholinesterase inhibitors and it seems these should be plainly noted on labels for arthritics. *(Nightshades are cholinesterase inhibitors which induce muscle stiffness, spasms.)*

"I plan to keep all nightshades out of my diet *forever* and hope to get it down to a fine point. It is so much trouble to carry out this Diet that I am afraid arthritic sufferers will not be able to successfully do the Diet, and realize the relief they so desire. What a shame! Also, I have been tempted to write food processors and explain my predicament hoping they may decide to omit the bell pepper or paprika or potato starch from at least some of their products, but I have not done it as I felt it would be hopeless. Some manufacturers put only "spices" on the label and these are suspect for paprika. Eating out is very difficult as the waitress always says, "How do you want your potato — mashed, baked or French fries?" And I pay through the nose for every slip! JR: Ala.
Note: This lady is 35 yrs., sports inclined, gardener, enjoys being a wife and housekeeper, and has been free of pain only a few days the past five years.

IN TIME I LEARNED TO ADHERE STRICTLY TO DIET

Fortunately for me, I read about your Diet for arthritis. It seemed nutty enough to be logical. After living with an aggravating case of tendinitis (viral, I was told) since 1945 and arthritis of the back and neck caused initially by two rear-end auto accidents, I decided to try your Diet. I had been going to the doctor 100x/yr or 3x/wk, was wearing an aggravating collar. At first, I eliminated the most obvious except where my desires overcame my common sense. In time, I have learned to adhere strictly to the Diet. After much experimenting, I have found I get reaction to even the minutest amounts of the nightshades. It just ain't worth it to eat any of them. No more aspirins, valium, motrin, or clinoril for me. Adhering to the Diet is all it takes and it *is* worth it! Thanks for helping me. SB:N.J.

DIET OR CHIROPRACTOR?

I have your book, decided to try the Diet over 9 mos. ago. Had just gotten out of the hospital with a two-week stay for severe arthritic problems and within a week I was back in trouble again. There was terrific pain in my left shoulder, neck and my hands were so badly swollen I could not make a fist, either hand. On the Diet my pains were much better after about two months. Could make fists and I was much more active than I could remember. I started going to a chiropractor twice weekly. Continued to improve but I am not certain which or both were doing it. But after a year of horrible pain and discomfort, I am not questioning which — I am a different person. Now, I seem to be something of a freak since this kind of recovery is rare. My former arthritic specialist says I am dealing with "quacks" so I tell him anyway they are good quacks. They solved my problem. My wife eats the same as I do now and has shown little improvement, but is still smoking cigarettes heavily. I am constantly being asked what happened to me! Several people want to contact you directly. My book is making the rounds among several of my arthritic friends. Thanks very much for the tremendous improvement I have made. DCA, Sr.:Md.

PIZZA, PORK AND BEANS

For many years, I have experienced pain and swelling in my knees and finger joints. When I cut out the two nightshades I eat regularly, potato and tomato, the result was noticeable almost immediately in my knees. Pain subsided in my finger joints. I have learned that a few French fries, a slice of pizza or pork and beans (tomato sauce) will bring painful reaction in my fingers overnight. Would you send me the complete diet? JDS:Ore.

SMOKING MAKES A DIFFERENCE

On the nightshade-free diet I feel much better. I can entertain more, drive more, even to Florida by myself, almost but not quite back to normal activities for me. Have not given up smoking yet, entirely. Quit twice, started twice! Stopping smoking is my next goal. And I find it does make a difference in my aches and pains. In my experience with pain killers, I found that aspirin does not cause a rash for me, but it does give minor gastro-intestinal bleeding. The Tylenol appears to give me dermatographia which is not a rash, but when I scratch my skin a red raised line appears. There is some itching. When I quit Tylenol, it took several weeks for this to go away. When I take a few Tylenol, the problem comes back and I never had it before taking this drug. I have been reading technical information in the media that says a high-protein diet may cause calcium to be taken from the bones and deposited in spurs. Is this true? *(No. But the nightshades will induce this. NFC).* I am so grateful to you for having the training and good sense to put your observations of your own well-being into a theory that has proven itself in helping so many people. HN:Wis.

BUMPER TOMATO CROP, EATING SOME, WILL STOP IF HURTS!

Note: This case was one of our first cooperators in 1975. She eventually became free of all pains and 4 years later had started trying a few tomatoes with no pains at last communication. Some people may be able to go back to eating a few nightshades without too much trouble, but each person will need to decide for himself if any pains developing are worth it. Under this condition some allergists claim that the nightshades are only an allergy to some people, but what is an allergy? We assume it is an undesirable reaction to something in the environment which is actually a poison to that particular person's body. Doctors say allergies come and go, but in our experience, this seems doubtful with the nightshades. You will note the lady below is eating tomatoes again but also gone back to taking a number of pills trying to correct "something". N.F.C.

"After 3½ years, it is time to write you about my progress. Really am free from pain. Still watching my diet closely. Even with a vacation and two weeks in the hospital, I can say it is great to feel good. It was a bit difficult at times but I came through alright. Here's hoping the other case histories have come through as good as I. Happy Holidays."

Note: The following summer, after 4 years, we received this evaluation on a survey reply card: "Somewhat on the Diet; taking iron, B_{12} and C vitamins, not smoking; eating tomatoes, a bumper crop, so far no effect, will discontinue if problems develop. Changed brand of C pills; they bothered me. I use C pills instead of sinus medicine. Right now no pain." MA:Ill.

PEPPER IN VITAMIN C PILLS

I receive three different catalogues that advertise vitamin C pills with peppers in them. In some bakery places, they use potato flour in breads, donuts, rolls, etc. I found out the hard way. Some breaded frozen products contain potato starch. Chocolate gives me migrain headaches. Too much coffee or tea upsets my stomach. Last fall I was tired too much of the time so went to the doctor and he gave me butazolidin pills, 100 mg. After two pills every joint in my body hurt, so I went back and he suggested vitamin B_{12} pills 500 mg 3x/wk. and they helped a lot. There is something in one brand of peanut butter; 3 hrs. after eating it I was in misery; could it have been paprika for flavoring; it was not indicated on the can. Outside of some of these things that sneak in, I have been pain-free and it is a wonderful feeling to be able to work in the garden and do all my housework with a lot of energy and no pain. My eyes had been deteriorating due to diabetes, but the doctor checked them after being on the Diet four months. He said there were no signs of further deterioration, or, in fact, no eye disease. IB:Ark.

Note: This lady is 52 yrs., had feet, hands, shoulders, knees, chest and back problems, was eating the nightshades, most of them almost daily, did not smoke. Most doctors told her to take aspirin, walk, use heat pads, and exercise. She had had the problems 25 yrs.

HAPPY HOLIDAY

"You have made my life so enjoyable because of your arthritic study that I had to wish you a "Happy Holiday". I have totally eliminated the nightshades from my diet and have no pain any more. I am a good detective at the grocery store and read all the labels for paprika, potato, tomato, etc. I do not take any drugs. My life is so much more pleasant. I wonder if the trauma of a divorce after 21 years could have brought on my arthritis. I am only 39 years old. Well, anyway, thanks!" E.J.:Ind. (Registered nurse).

HAVEN'T FELT SO GOOD IN YEARS!

I am 54 and have had arthritic problems for 22 yrs. My fingers are puffy, swollen at the knuckles and most of the aches and pains are in my feet and hands with some problem in my ankles, knees, hips and elbows. I have eaten the nightshades all my life and regularly. I smoke Kent cigarettes and am taking 10-12 aspirins a day which give only temporary relief. Walking is painful. I felt better within 3 mos. of going on the Diet but I had a few flareups from peppers and paprika hidden in foods. My husband and I read ingredients on containers carefully now. Chocolate has bothered me some. My problem has been smoking but I have cut down considerably and can see the difference. I have been on the diet for almost two years now and want to say that the Diet has helped me tremendously. I know it works, having gone off the Diet a few times, but get right back to avoid continuing hurts. I have even gotten myself a part time job which really pleases me. Thank you so much for your help. Note my change of address. LMH:Ind.

93 AND ON THE DIET WITHOUT KNOWING IT!

Thinking back over my childhood, I find something that had not been given much thought. My childhood was spent with many relatives and a lot of different people. One aunt who lived to be 93 and never had any signs of arthritis seemed to be on the diet without knowing it. She lived on the Gulf Coast. There we had rice and grits frequently and our "potatoes" were actually *sweet potatoes.* We never saw an eggplant. Tomatoes, a few, were used in season.

I now have been on the Diet for three months and here are the results: (1) Better balance; (2) lack of stiffness; (3) finger on right hand next to little finger nearly straight; (4) much more agility; (5) much less bloated feeling; (6) better digestion; and (7) generally better health. Incidentally, I am enclosing a catalogue description of a combination of potato, tomato and pepper in one plant, the tomato and pepper grafted onto a potato I assume, for about $6 from a nursery in Hanover, Pa. My gosh, what are they going to do to us next! MGM:NM. (See "Toe-peperatoe" photograph in Chap. I.)

SEND SOME BROCHURES

Enclosed is money for another copy of your book. Please send some brochures for my friends. A lot of people around here are interested in this Diet. I became aware through a friend whose entire family had great results, faith in and praise for your book! JK:Wa.

WEATHER MAKES NO DIFFERENCE NOW!

It has been 16 months since I discontinued the nightshades and 10 months since I stopped vitamin pills. The results have been very good. It took at least 6 months before noticeable results. And stopping the vitamin pills made even more improvement. I agree that an occasional flareup in my knee is due to a nightshades intake without my being aware. I continue to read labels before purchasing or cooking. My favorite Planters Roasted Peanuts have paprika on them so I had to eliminate them from my snacks. I have been without pain and swelling in my fingers for months and months regardless of the weather conditions. Thanks for your Newsletter. I shall continue my vigil on labels! BB:Ohio

Note: BB was 53 yrs., eating nightshades regularly and heavily, had two discs removed from spine, causing use of traction when all other treatments failed; previously sprained wrist a problem. Gave up eating chocolate and yogurt every day, feet hurt badly, she "won't give up"! Stopped a sleeping pill that had scopolamine (nightshade) in it.

"HOW ABOUT THAT QUACK, DR. FREDERICKS?

Note: The author gets calls frequently from this area regarding weekday nightly programs of Dr. Carleton Fredericks, well known to his millions of listeners over the USA and Canada (programs are taped and sent to many USA stations). In a recent call, a husband was urged by his wife to eall that Dr. Childers at Rutgers University and see if the suggestions of Dr. Carleton Fredericks (that "quack", as noted by her doctor) on WOR, New York City, is correct about the nightshades and arthritis. She had been told by her doctor, that "there is absolutely no relation between diet and arthritis." I relisted the foods involved and apparently the caller had been eating them every day, for his reply was, "Yes, and those are my favorite foods", indicating at the end of the conversation that he had severe problems and would try the Diet.

Dr. Fredericks has been on radio and TV WOR for over 35 yrs. His main theme has been the relation between diet, drugs and health and sickness of people, both physically and mentally. He is a PhD and notes this fact often on his programs for the A.M.A. has tried many times to remove him from the air, but unsuccessfully due to his millions of loyal listeners. He also gets hundreds of letters from his periodic references to the No-Nightshades Childers' Diet, and reads them on the air. N.F. Childers.

MULTIPLE SCLEROSIS AND ?

I am 51, 120 lbs, had arthritis in knees and back for 8 yrs, but was diagnosed in Barnes Hospital, St. Louis, in 1959 as having MS. But it seems to me there is a question among doctors on diagnosis and cures for MS. Your book has convinced me that hanging a name on a disease does not mean too much. A disease is a disease. My symptoms were loss of balance, numbness about the jaw and mouth, and nystagmus (rolling eyeballs). My hearing was affected, None of the problems persisted after the first attack. Eight years ago I started going down hill again and Yoga and a special diet helped in which I did not repeat foods day after day, switched around. But my knees and back were bad and I found that the No-Nightshades Diet helped my back and also stopped headaches and fever. I have great hope for you and our Diet in curing many diseases. My husband would rather have his aches and pains than give up potatoes and tomatoes and I only buy them when he insists. Is that fair to him? Incidentally, peanuts are bad for me. PK:Mo.

Note: We need more information on MS, Myasthenia Gravis, glaucoma, nervous disorders, others as they may be related to the Nightshades. We would appreciate hearing from you or working with you if you have one of these problems. The nightshades are undoubtedly related to many unsolved diseases. NFC.)

EXCELLENT RESULTS (ITALIAN LADY)

"I have been on the Diet for over a year now and am very grateful to report excellent results. I don't even take aspirin which I had taken in heavy quantities for 10 years. I am now pain-free with little or no morning stiffness unless I cheat on the Diet (I have a weakness for pizza). I am now smoking "lights" and trying hard to cut that out, but it is very difficult. I have no swelling in my hands but do have nodes on my index fingers and thumb. I am considering undergoing corrective surgery. I have had such a total response that word has spread among friends and one older lady was in such pain that even medication could not alleviate it. Today I spoke with her husband and she is pain-free — without pills and within 3 months! Thank you, thank you — the word is spreading fast." G.S.P.:Me.

"YOU'll NEVER IMPROVE" — MD

"I began the Diet almost a year ago. Results excellent. M.D. said I'd never improve. He cannot believe I am off medication. I've passed information on to several friends with your address." T.L.S.:Ga.

Note: Man is 60 years, had problems 5 years, 172 lbs., travel 75%, "cheaters" or hidden "sneakers" cause problem, so must watch carefully; no problem to eliminate obvious nightshades.

MAN STANDING ON CHEST NO MORE!

"Before the Diet I had a problem sitting in church when all of a sudden it felt like a man standing on my chest — hard to breathe. Now there is no pain down my left arm, chest has cleared, ankles and feet are fine, walk straight, no elbow or back problems. One afternoon I felt I had to eat the hostess' eggplant parmesan and that night the pain was horrible in my back and at the base of my spine. It hurt all the next day. I could hardly get out of a chair. I was amazed that just a little eggplant could do that to me so quickly." R.S.D.:Fla.
Note: This lady is 72, smokes occasionally, is completely free of aches and pains that used to make her limp and limited her walking.

FROM PUERTO RICO

"Fifth and 6th vertebrae diagnosed as causing pain in left shoulder and arm and could not write with left hand, thought to be caused by driving on bad roads for several years. Skin rash controlled by avoiding hexachlorophenol. Astounding improvement in three months on Diet. No pains except infrequently when probably got a nightshade inadvertently. Had to work at the Diet to perfect it, but it was worth it. I am now able to write again without any effort." J.H.C., P.R.

POTATOES FOR LIVESTOCK FEED?

Due to drouth this year potato farmers had a "cull" crop, so Federal Aid is permitting the farmers to spread out the potatoes on frozen fields, then pick them up frozen next spring and ship them to livestock farmers for feed. My question is about the meat and milk from these livestock. Will the solanine, etc., be in the milk and meat? (Answer: probably a little but we need research here. It is probable that the solanine will increase with long exposure of the potatoes to light). We want to eat our potatoes since we grew them and we do hate to throw them out. If we feed them to our hens, will it hurt us to eat the eggs and chickens. *(Answer: we cannot be sure, maybe).*

Up here in northern Aroostook, Maine there are many retarded children. Now most farmers ship out their best potatoes and eat the blighted and culls. Just a thought. The three of us in this family were tomato growers in Massachusetts before moving here (Note: they are now back in Mass.) We all have arthritis rather badly. Could it have been from not only eating the tomatoes but trying to get the yellow-green stain off our hands after working with the plants? We took steel wool and a brush to try to get it off. *(Answer: yes, the chemicals very likely entered the blood stream through the skin since we know that nicotine sulphate, used for insect control from tobacco, will enter the skin and make people sick if they get too much of the spray drift.)* Just questions to help. We are in this with our whole heart. MB:Mass.

PLEASE. MORE INFORMATION

My husband read a short item about the No-Nightshades Diet in the local paper last November and stopped eating the nightshades. Six months later he is completely free of pains and aches. Our friends are getting interested. Please send us a book, or reprint, or something more about the Diet. We are in a senior citizen development. HD:Ariz.

Recently a friend of mine sent a short article from Alaska about the nightshades. I am 76 and have had severe swelling in my right knee. I eliminated the nightshades and I hardly use my cane any more. Please send me more information on the diet. My doctors have told me there is no relation between diet and arthritis and I have heard this many years since I fell and had three surgeries on the knee. LC: Wa.

An R. N. friend shared a news article about the nightshades with me and I eliminated the four vegetables. I had great discomfort in arms, elbows and shoulders. In three weeks I am completely free of aches and pains. Is it possible? Please send more information. GFM:Wa.

89 YEARS YOUNG — JUST FINE!

This emeritus professor who brought artificial insemination of dairy cattle to the USA and wrote a book about it, had arthritic problems but was very skeptical about the Diet, since his best friend was an emeritus professor of vegetable gardening. But two years after starting the Diet, he says, "I could not straighten out my little right finger on arising in the morning. By working with it, finally it would loosen up. My hip was bad too. Since early last November that digital trouble has entirely disappeared. I also play golf with no trouble, more durability. My knee hurts a little and I shall have to cut way back on the chocolate since that is the only No-No I have been eating." (He received an honorary doctorate from Rutgers University, 1980). EP:N.J.

NOW I BUY SMALLEST ASPIRIN BOTTLE

Just a line to let you know I feel 300% better now since going on the Diet. Instead of buying the largest bottle of aspirin I now buy the smallest, and only take them once in a while. I used to live on them. If I ride the bicycle a lot, I may have to take an aspirin at night, but only one. I am very grateful to have found out about the No-Nightshades Diet. I am 53 and had arthritis all over. I went to a specialist who just told me to take aspirin, that I had arthritis and "did not know how to grow old gracefully." I have not been back since inasmuch as I know myself I have a lot of pains and could hardly walk. I was furious. I intend to stay on this Diet forever. JAS:Ca.

HANDS COLD, BONES "FROZEN"

I have had diagnosed rheumatoid arthritis since the 1950s and the doctor told me nothing could be done about it. As the years went by my hands got worse. I could not knit without pain and I cannot tell you the horrible thoughts that used to go through my mind. My cousin read an article about your work and I immediately went on the diet which is painless and very economical. I used to eat a lot of the nightshade vegetables. After 6 mos., my hands now are so straight, thinned down, and feel on the inside just great. They used to feel like the bones were frozen they were so cold. I now can make a tight fist, knit and do everything without pain. I also have been doing yoga daily and exercise them often. I work in a store and do some typing and writing also.

From the bottom of my heart, I want to thank you so very much for this information. Thanks, thanks, thanks.I have your book too. Have a good Thanksgiving and you can be sure I shall have one too! CJ:N.J.

CRIPPLING IN ITALY

I have suffered from arthritis ever since I was in my teens and was living in northern Italy, where potatoes and tomatoes are the main foods consumed daily. Incidentally, while revisiting that region recently, I noticed that nearly all of its natives in their mid and upper years are suffering from crippling arthritis.

For the past 10 yrs. I have avoided the tomato after extensive allergy tests and the pain in my knees decreased somewhat intermittently. Meantime, the pain in my finger joints became more intense. I was desperate when last November I read in Prevention magazine about the toxicity of the nightshades for the first time. From that time, I eliminated *all* the nightshades, together with hot spices. By Christmas the pain in my fingers had completely subsided.

The veracity of your findings was proven again recently when, while spending a week in Texas and Mexico, I was not able entirely to avoid tomatoes, hot peppers and sauces, especially in my favorite food, shrimps. The pain in my fingers returned and still bothers me two weeks later. I do not smoke and haven't for 30 yrs.

Dr. Childers, I wish I could help you in educating people about the toxicity of the nightshades. I am thoroughly convinced. You are right in saying that it is not difficult to find alternatives for the pervasive and pernicious potato. Incidentally, even the ancient Peruvian Indians suffered from arthritis, according to anthropologists and historians, and they were heavy potato eaters and still are. The potato originated in Peru. *(My Peace Corp students working in Peru tell me the Peruvian life span in the mountains is only 25-30 yrs. NFC).* Thank you, Dr. Childers, for helping me and best of luck in your worthwhile efforts to help others. YAC:Wis.

ONLY EIGHT SALTED ALMONDS (WITH PAPRIKA)!

After 3 mos. on the Diet, I have more pep, and a few days with pain. My sore heel is almost totally gone. But last week I ate 8 salted almonds and found later they had paprika on them. For two days after I was miserable. Could it have been the paprika on only 8 almonds? Is this possible? How can we spread the word faster, other than telling our friends? Could we tell something of your findings to *The National Enquirer,* or is the paper "too far out"? I wish arthritics everywhere could know about the Diet! DED:Wa.

NEW IDEAS ARE RIDICULED, LAUGHED AT AND DAMNED!

After reading your book on Nightshades I am more convinced about the connection between this family of plants and arthritis. I'd like to see a carefully conducted survey with ethnic groups of people to see if those in the Mediterranean area and Ireland who are unusually large users of the nightshade plants, would have more health problems, particularly arthritis and crippling. Also, make a survey of the same groups among the Americans. As I told you in an earlier letter, you will find great resistance from farmers, processors, doctors, drug manufacturers and even the Arthritis Foundation to your approach to arthritis control. Others before you with new ideas have been ridiculed, laughed at and damned! If you and your partner are correct, you certainly should have a double Nobel prize. *PP:PhD., N.Y.*

CHEESE PROBLEM

I have been on the Diet for 4 months, and after receiving your book, found there were some things to avoid that were not in the magazine article. I quit 1000 mg Vitamin C daily and my nausea went away. By Christmas, I could actually turn over in bed which I hadn't been able to do for a long time. But we bought a large 5 lb. round of cheese (cheddar) and I decided to try eating it every day to see if I felt a difference. In less than a wk. I could scarcely turn over in bed or get up out of a rocking chair (probably paprika). It took almost a month to get back to where I was in recovery. I am following the Diet to the utmost and using only a small amount of milk in cooking — no fresh milk (build-up of Vitamin D). I sent the clipping from Organic Gardening to my cousin in Texas who also has been on the Diet four months. He could not walk without a limp and could not reach his arms above his head. By Thanksgiving he did not limp and could easily raise his arms high and continues to see improvement every week. There is no comparison how I feel now and when I started the Diet! I broke my hand two months ago and my doctor is amazed that arthritis did not settle in it. Mrs. ETC: Okla.

Note: This lady is 65 yrs., 134 lbs., had hysterectomy for small uterus cancer, was taking numerous pain killers, having muscle spasms, headaches and a back problem.

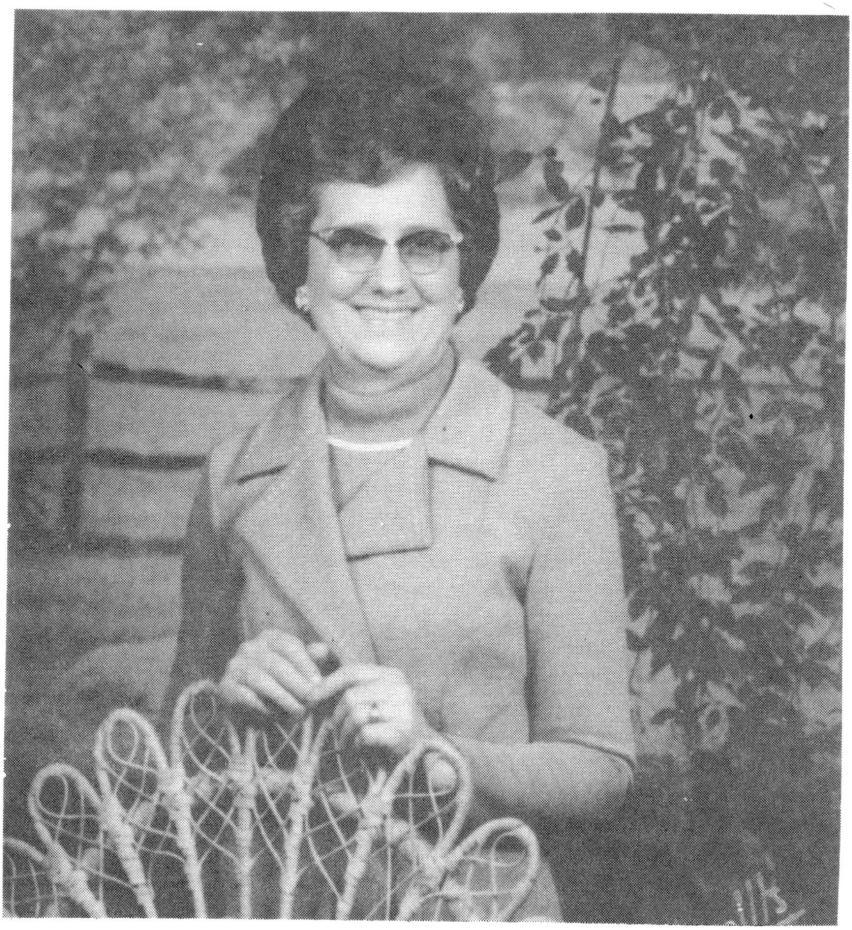

Mrs. Harold N. (Georgia) Cross
Lexington, Tennessee
"I shall never again eat them. Now I can do anything I want to."

'I SHALL NEVER AGAIN EAT THEM'

Since May I have been omitting the nightshade plants and their products from my diet, and I am thrilled with the results. I'm so much better that I shall never again eat them.

Before the diet, my knees hurt, as did my back, elbows, neck, shoulder and ankles. My hands hurt so much I could hardly do my housework (they tingled and the fingers of my left hand were numb — I could hardly hold a dish). I could not move my wrist because of the pain. And I could only brush my hair by holding the back of the brush, not the handle.

I still have pains in my fingers and knees at times, and my fingers are stiff when I first get up in the morning. But my hands are no longer numb and I can dust without pain — I have no trouble at all.

LUPUS

"I have been diagnosed as having lupus (a form of arthritis). Since on this Diet for about one month I have not suffered any aches and pains whereas before I had very bad aches. I am reducing my cortisone from 60 to 40 and now to 15 mg/wk." DL:N.J.

Note: This Italian girl was 23 yrs. at start, 110 lbs., problem 3 yrs., sensitive to light, skin rash, slight hair loss, joints swollen and aching, in feet, knees, elbows, shoulders, neck, lower back; ate potatoes, tomatoes, ketchup daily. We have a few other cooperators with lupus who have or are recovering; we would appreciate hearing from others. She had tried many doctors, last one said "diet not a factor"; all doctors wanted to medicate, their only approach to relief. NFC.

ARTHRITIS AND TOBACCO, FARM WORK?

I read about your theory and eliminated the nightshades from my diet since the past year I started getting stiffness in my joints. It worked — no stiffness any more, except when I go back to potato or tomato. I had always avoided tomatoes until this year when we started growing them in our garden. My aunt has been severely afflicted with arthritis for many years; she lives on a tobacco farm. Is it conceivable that being around tobacco and working with it, could cause symptoms of arthritis without it actually being ingested? She does not use tobacco *(Yes. Plant chemicals can be absorbed through the skin by handling the fruits and the plant.)*

HANDS BETTER FOR GARDENING, PAINTING

Please send me more information about the Diet you have. I read about it in a Health Digest magazine, omitted the nightshades from my diet and found that it does lessen the arthritis in my hands. I now can enjoy watering hundreds of plants in my garden again and when I work at my painting, the brushes do what I hope they will! MS:N.J.

NEWS TO ME — NIGHTSHADES AND ARTHRITIS!

I read about this theory in Organic Gardening and eliminated these vegetables from my diet and within this short time of three months have found a big change in the use of my hands, hips and shoulders. I have had joint trouble for over 20 yrs. and have tried about everything with the usual ups and downs of pain. Nowhere have I ever heard of the nightshade vegetables causing arthritis. In my case, the elimination of the dearly beloved tomato and potato were well worth it. No difficulty in eliminating the other nightshades. HDR:Mi.

WHOLE FAMILY RESPONDED

We started the Diet about 3 months ago, wife 37, daughter 8½ and me, 45 yrs. We ate a lot of ketchup, French fries, etc. My wife and daughter have had rheumatism in their knees nearly all their lives. (My wife is from Tahati). No pains anymore. And my wife's facial condition has much improved. My joints still are a little stiff at times but much improved and I have a lot more muscle strength — can lift a 100 lb. bag of cement with no trouble at all, whereas it used to be a real strain! I was surprised at this. No chronic chest congestion now. Also, no more popping, swelling across second knuckle when close hand to a fist. *(His last letter says they are continuing to improve every month over almost 2 yrs.)* NKS:Mo.

DELIBERATELY WENT OFF DIET

As a cooperator, I want to tell you I deliberately went off the diet and had tomatoes, potatoes and peppers. The end result — pains returned to foot and ankle. It just ain't worth the pains! I try to stay with the Diet rigidly but occasionally something slips in without me being aware of it — and I learn it the next day or two. I have told many friends about the diet and some are now trying it. So glad I heard about the diet from a friend and sent for the book. RCD: N.J.

SUGGESTED DIET TO MY PATIENTS

Please forward more information about your Diet. I saw the note in Organic Gardening and suggested the omission of these foods from the diet of several of my patients and the results are GREAT. Thank you very much for this research. Dr. GHD: Mo. (Chiropractor)

MAY TAKE TWO YEARS.

This is the 6th month I have followed your instructions with the aid of my wife. I wish to report: (1) My stamina has increased a lot; (2) I am able to do yard work, painting, and many other tasks that were almost impossible before; (3) The swelling in my hands is completely gone; (4) I sleep from 10 P.M. to 6 A.M. now every night; (5) The total pains have certainly lessened but I do still have some. But I am discouraged since you said it may take two years to best a long-standing problem. GES:Ca.

TOOK 24 BUFFERINS A DAY

My husband can't hardly see to write, so I shall do it. He is so thrilled about your book, "Nightshades and Health" that he tells everyone about the nightshades. He is thrilled about what the Diet has done for him. He used to take 24 bufferins a day, 6 at a time, he had so much pain. His joints are no longer stiff. He walks with a spring again. He used to smoke 2½ packs of cigarettes a day but since his heart attack last fall, he is down to ½ pack, trying to stop completely. We thank you so much and wish you the best. EAC:NV

CAN'T FORECAST WEATHER ANY MORE!

I read about the No-Nightshades Diet in the Rutgers Alumni Monthly and switched from aspirin to the diet. I have taken aspirin for 20 years, tried all the doctor's remedies, even acupuncture, and was thinking about trying Clinoril. After one month on the diet, my constant aches and pains in my neck, shoulders, hands, knees and back have all but disappeared. I no longer put double wrappings on my knees at night before bed, nor woolen gloves on my hands. It seems my only loss is that I can no longer forecast the weather change by my aching knees. Must go back to the barometer! Bless you for your discovery. SL:N.J.

I'M A PIANIST, TYPIST, ARTIST — NEED NIMBLE FINGERS!

My hands are so important to me, being a pianist, typist, artist and organist. Aspirin helps to loosen my fingers, but not enough. Your Diet program has been very helpful to me. My pains and stiffness are much less, but on a vacation — they all came back and it took awhile to get back to no stiffness and pain. Avoiding these foods is really working for me. Please keep me on your mailing list. AB:S.C.

RATHER TAKE PILLS!

I am very grateful for the help I am getting from the Diet. I have been doing what I can to spread the word. Sad to say, most folks "don't hear me"! I've loaned the book to many, but they are not serious about the Diet. *One friend told me she would rather take pills. Incredible!* I have been on the diet a year and also took off 50 lbs and had thought perhaps this could be the main reason for feeling better. So I started eating potato, paprika, etc. Return — the pains and stiffness. Spinach bothers my husband and me, seems to cause hives. We also have reduced intake of sugar. It is amazing how many things contain potato, tomato and paprika. I have started cooking most of our food to be sure. This summer I have been walking, running, riding my bike, doing anything and everything without pain. I am not about to eat the No-Nos again! DED:Wash.

"EAT ANYTHING YOU WISH!"

I know arthritis can be helped with diet. I've done it, but, in so doing, made mistakes — potatoes, my weakness. I was following Dr. Dong's Diet and did improve but still had problems til I found your book. He had potatoes and eggplant in his diet. I couldn't pull my coat or clothes over my left arm, and now I can. My body is free from *all* pain. Doctors have told me, "Eat anything you wish, diet has no relation to arthritis." In fact, The Foundation emphasizes this. I shall be on this Diet as long as I live! Here is $100 to help with your work. RH: NV.

REGISTERED NURSE RESPONDED

I am 55 yrs., an R.N., 135 lbs., have had rheumatoid arthritis for 7 years, but have had joint pains since 7 yrs. old with times of remission. I have tried numerous pain killers, other treatments but this Diet has me feeling much better. I went off the Diet for 2 wks. with the old problems coming back so I'm on the Diet again and back to "normal". Problems were in my feet, ankles, hands, and chest. ELS:Ma.

WINTER WEATHER NOT A FACTOR; CAN SLEEP NOW.

I have been on the No-Nightshades Diet for 6 mos. and am fully convinced the nightshades do affect painful muscles and joints. I feel much better. Our hard Wyoming winter with 20-30°F below zero day after day did not cause any increase in aches and pains so evidently the Diet is the answer. I got through the winter in fine health. Feet, hip, hands and knee pains all gone and I enjoy increased vitality, durability and sound sleep.

Two months ago I started taking Rose Hip vitamin C, thinking there would be no nightshades C in it, but the joint on my right thumb swelled and was as painful as a boil. So within two days after stopping these pills, the swelling went down, no pains. Now I get my "C" from fruits and vegetables. I am so thankful I know about this Diet and, actually, I do not miss nightshades in the menus. LMP: Wyo.

82 YRS, DISCARDED MY CANE

I live alone at a retired village and am interested in living comfortably as long as I can. I have listened to you on Dr. Frederick's WOR New York City Station and read about you in the "Experienced Citizen". I was quite crippled, lumps on ankle, knee, hip and shoulders and have had to use a cane until recently. My doctor tried all the drugs on me that my neighbors are taking, but I could not get them all to stay down. So then my doctor advised I do as he said at the start and take only aspirin continually — pain or no pain, and to take it with milk. I told my doctor about your approach of eliminating the tomato, potato, peppers and eggplant and he told me if I did that to replace with his suggested foods so I would not suffer from mineral deficiencies, etc. Well, after a month or so on your Diet, I had no aches or pains. But in August the following when my favorite vegetable, tomato, was in season, I started eating them and baked potatoes too. In September I had a seizure of those terrible pains again, so no more of the nightshades. I have finished for life all those things you mention and I am very grateful to you. I have had some bad pains in my life but nothing so miserable as arthritis pains. For a long time I had to use a cane, but no longer, thank you, thank you. I shall write to the Arthritis Foundation in the hopes that they will use this Diet to help the thousands of sufferers all over the country. ECH:N.J.

"YOU MUST LEARN TO LIVE WITH PAINS!"

I am 56 yrs., 140 lbs. and have had osteoarthritis for over 20 yrs. mainly in my back, but also problems in my knees, hips, elbows and neck. Plus skin rashes. I took butazolidin until I became allergic to it, then pains in back were constant with muscle spasms in my legs every day. After reading the item in Organic Gardening about the nightshades I ceased eating them but it took about a year to really see differences. My whole back feels better, I sleep better, my fingers are returning to normal size, and I never have leg cramps anymore, or muscle spasms. The symptoms return when I eat at restaurants and try potatoes and tomatoes again with a little paprika on fish. I don't take vitamin pills very often, although I did take heavy doses under a doctor's direction and he also told me, "You must learn to live with pains!" LN:Ore.

ORANGE PEEL OIL A PROBLEM?

In regard to vitamin C pills causing sore feet and enlarged joints, we do know in our experience that orange peel oil and "C" pills from some natural sources (with paprika?) will cause irritation and rash in some patients. Considering the useful information in your book, I think the price is very reasonable ($20). RB:Ca., M.D.

"ASKING MY PATIENTS TO COOPERATE WITH YOU"

Congratulations on a bit of detective work — I have your nightshades book. I intend to put this to use with as many of my patients as it seems applicable. If you have any kind of study cards, I shall give them to my patients and ask them to complete them and return to you. *Note: In later correspondence several of the doctor's patients have shown marked improvement as noted in clippings sent fom Prevention Magazine).* JVW:Wa., M.D.

FLUID IN KNEES — 25 YEARS OLD

"I am only 25 years old but have had a severe problem with arthritis for a long time. I loved tomatoes. Ate them voraciously. My mother got me off tomatoes and now I am 100% better. I can walk, drive a car, play volleyball. When we read your article in Organic Gardening, I was very pleased that someone is working on this problem and doing some good to help us sufferers. The pain was so bad before going on the Diet, I had to hold onto a table to sit down, had to fight just to stay conscious when climbing the stairs, the pain was so bad and my knees were often filled with fluid. I haven't taken aspirin in over a year. I did not want to do the Diet but my mom practically made me, so the results are "not just in my head"! I thank the Lord you discovered this thing! I have a few friends just starting the Diet and they will write to you." L.M.R.:Ky.

OTHER DISEASES RESPOND TO DIET.

We have been very interested in the No-Nightshades Diet and have had several patients who have had complete remission of symptoms within one week after starting the Diet . . . We find that citrus and grains may cause allergies in some people and milk is the cause of gastrointestinal, skin, and emotional problems. We would add to your list of diseases corrected by the nightshades Diet: Menopause, thyroid problems, colitis, peptic ulcers and the hypoglycemic syndrome. We appreciate your efforts in this field and thanks for putting us on your mailing list. AMY:Ala.-M.D.

MAYBE I CAN HELP WITH RESEARCH FUNDS

(Phone call from California). I am a dentist, 65 yrs, formerly lived in South Jersey, and we hear Dr. Carleton Fredericks often — about 5 minutes each morning and he gives us more news on human nutrition than it is possible to get anywhere. He told us about your Diet and I am inquiring for myself and another lady who visits my office for dental work who is restricted by arthritis. I have watched my daughter peel and cut tomatoes and her eyes will tear and her nose drip. My nose responds similarly. Hence, I am wondering if I might be one of the 70% + who will respond to the Diet. Incidentally, I am in contact with people who try to find places to put their money and I am going to suggest your research as a worthy project. I understand you are establishing a Foundation for this purpose . . . Good luck, you will hear from me. EVP:Ca. DDS.

I GET PLENTY TO EAT WITHOUT NIGHTSHADES

I just had to sit down and tell you about the results with your No-Nightshades Diet. I am 74 yrs, 180 lbs, walk for exercise, do not smoke, and have diverticulitis. I have been on the diet for over 6 months. I had bad pains in my knees and leg the past 3 yrs. I had to take both hands to get my leg in bed a little at a time the pain was so bad. I needed help in and out of a car and I walked with a cane. Two doctors suggested surgery but I declined and decided to suffer the pain. After hearing about your Diet, I began avoiding the nightshades. About three weeks ago I got up in the morning with *no pain* and could not believe it. I now can lift my leg in bed without help, can get in and out of cars by myself, walk without a cane. I have been very faithful to the Diet and find that I get all the food I want without the nightshades. My senior citizen friends say they can see a big differenc in my facial expressions (without the pain). I have loaned my book to several friends. I cannot tell you how glad I am to have heard about your Diet. MC:N.J.

DISTANT VISION NOW GREAT: SPREADING THE WORD.

Thanks for last Newsletter — I am *so* happy to be among the fortunate 72% + with positive results. At this point I do not use any prepared foods, except once in awhile cheese, bread and canned fruit. I watch all labels carefully, as you have instructed. For years I have enjoyed a small glass of brandy, perhaps 2 to 3 times a yr. I find now that this seems to set off pains and stiffness, so I avoid it. I follow your instructions to a "T". I am now able to hike, ride my bike (at 66 yrs, 175 lbs), mow the grass, work in the yard, etc. with real comfort. I take no medicine — not even aspirin. I have told this story, written it, shouted it all across the country — in airports, on planes, in the beauty shops, in restrooms, everywhere, to friends and hundreds of strangers I never saw before. Would you believe it? Two of my best friends are miserable with arthritis, but I simply cannot get them to even try the Diet. Since I am able to take a good brisk walk every day, I am able to control my weight better, my circulation is better and hence, my distant vision is much better — great, in fact. Thank you, sir. I may never see you, but you are surely my finest friend. DD:Wa.

AND YOU APOLOGIZE FOR PRICE OF BOOK!

I am 63, heavy — 250 lbs, had problems for 6 yrs. Following your advice means I can take off a coat, comb my hair and scratch my back without pain. And you apologize for the price of the book! The advice in your book is worth many times its price. I wish I were in a financial condition that would let me contribute to your work but I am on a small pension and social security is all I have. I used to dread to go to sleep at night because I would roll over on my side (either side) and the pain would wake me up. I couldn't even comb my hair without bending my head over so I couldn't reach it. I could raise my arm only so high. My left thigh would ache until I took aspirin.

Now I'm building my own retirement home, handling heavy lumber, big sheets of plywood, climbing ladders and a thousand and one things entailed in building a home. All of the nightshades with the exception of tobacco which I gave up about 20 yrs ago, were my favorite foods. A stew without potatoes and green bell peppers — no way! Spaghetti sauce without tomatoes — heavens no. Eggplant, I'd have once in awhile. Well, I don't use any of them anymore except by mistake and when I buy canned food without reading the labels. But I'm soon aware of it with return of the aches. Enclosed is $10 to further your work . . . . I do wish it could be more but it is all I can spare. And from the very bottom of my heart, thank you. NB:N.Y.

EATS POTATOES, TOMATOES TIL BACK ACHES, THEN STOPS

At your suggestion we have no eggplant, peppers or pepper in the house, but my husband loves potatoes and tomatoes. If he eats large quantities of potatoes and tomatoes, he has a sleepless nite due to an aching back. And it will last for several days. Sometimes a stiff shoulder or ankle goes along with the back problem. He is willing to say now after several trials, that he can control his back ache by avoiding potatoes and tomatoes. John, at his fairly young age, thinks he can control back ache by the amount of tomatoes and potatoes he eats and is going by this philosophy now. These foods seem almost addicting to him — he just cannot imagine giving them up, but eventually he may have to. JH:NC.

I PREPARE OWN FOODS TO AVOID NIGHTSHADES

I am 64, 180 lbs, have had a hands, back and bad knees problem for 3 yrs. I never smoked. I go to the health spa and took Trilisate. I have been on the Diet about 1½ yrs. The numbness, itching in my hands, and the painful swollen joints do not bother me any more. X-rays show my left leg with bad knee is ¼ inch shorter than right leg, so doctor has given me a shoe lift. I had a tomato sandwich and the itching started again. I highly recommend the Diet to anyone with arthritis. "Go on it and stay on it"! I fix most of my foods in the home to avoid nightshades — bake bread, season my dishes, etc. NDM:Va.

BREAKTHROUGH IN YOUR BACKYARD!
(A Letter To A Newspaper)

The Courier-News (Somerville, N.J.) missed the boat last week by publishing Dr. Fries' (from California) five-part series on arthritis. You have in your own backyard (speaking to the Courier-News) Dr. Norman F. Childers, horticulturist at Rutgers University, who has made a significant breakthrough both in alleviating and curing people who have suffered for years with the crippling effects of this disease.

Dr. Fries' misconceptions and contradictions are appalling.

After 15 years of suffering from arthritis, Dr. Childers proved the effectiveness of the Diet (of no-nighthsades — no tomatoes, white potatoes, eggplant, tobacco, and peppers of all kinds except black pepper). His theory has helped this writer, her uncle who had the disease for 18 yrs, as well as another resident of Somerset County I know who threw away her crutches by following the Diet. This method costs nothing and thousands of collaborators are living proof that it works.

Dr. Childers deserves a Nobel Prize for relieving unnecessary human suffering.

Where else but from California does sexuality enter into the picture? FM:N.J.

Note: There was an item in the Messenger-Gazette paper appearing previously to the Courier-News items which told about the lady discarding her crutches. Then the five series items appeared in the Courier-News apparently sponsored by the Arthritis Foundation. Then this letter appeared which is typical over the country of numerous heated discussions about the Diet. NFC.

CAN CHALLENGE HUSBAND AGAIN — "YOUNG, ACTIVE!"

I must report on my continuing recovery from arthritis (at least, so-called). I am beginning to believe it is rather a "condition" caused by properties in foods we eat, as is so plainly explained in your book. The recovery of my whole body has been nothing less than remarkable (on Diet 2 yrs.), and almost unbelievable. My husband and I are equally enthusiastic about the book and the results, as we were both very concerned over my health. We hope you never run out of your book, as we would hope everyone so-afflicted would have opportunity to examine it and follow directions, if they so desire. We recommend it to everyone that will listen and have loaned our 2 copies to so many folks that we have lost count. These days I feel so good! I can even get down on my knees again! And with no pain or restriction — that was my last hurdle. I had always felt and acted young but for awhile there I almost believed I was getting OLD. Ha, that's all changed again, and I can even give my husband a challenge at "being young and active". I always had to push to keep up with him. I praise and thank the Lord for you and your work and others who also have the concern to get to the core of health problems, and not just to mask them by giving medications, etc. which really only make matters worse. God knows, we don't need that. Keep it up, and keep speaking out! With so many people hurting, they need help badly. God bless you. Thankfully, RR:Pa.

TOSSED THE CANE, ON THE BIKE NOW!

I am 56 yrs, 160 lbs., had problems for about 2 yrs, arthritis bad in knees, hands and elbows. I read your book about 2 yrs ago, sorry to be slow in answering. I quit the nightshades immediately and find the Diet really helps me. I am walking much better and not using a cane any more. I still have some aches but nothing like they were in the beginning which was about 6 months after a bad fall. I feel great and am riding my bike on the Ocean City Boardwalk. TAB:N.J.

WE NEED DIET RECIPES!

I was 76 yrs, double hip problem, one hip since replaced, other was said to be as bad but I objected. Now after 14½ months on your Diet, I am free of medication, riding my bike 5 miles a day, feeling fine. I had acupuncture, therapy exercises, doctor told me to take 12 aspirins a day, the whole bit. My wife and I have faithfully followed the Diet and I am definitely a "late bloomer". She has had considerable lessening of pain in her hands she has had since 1940. Both of us appreciate all that you have done in spreading the word with your Diet. I wish in the next edition of your book you would include a number of recipes — we need a real good vegetable soup or a Manhatten clam chowder made with a tomato substitute. You have a big roster of enthusiastic followers in this whole area. A set of good recipes would encourage more complete compliance with the Diet: GAE:N.J.

(Note: If you have a good recipe(s), send it to us for publication in the next edition. You will find some Diet recipes in Chapter II.

ARTHRITIS ALWAYS WORSE IN FALL AFTER SUMMER FLING

I have had rheumatoid arthritis since 19 yrs of age and am now 38. I first saw your diet in Prevention magazine and realized that my aches and pains were always worse in the fall after eating nightshades voraciously from my garden and roadside stands. I don't smoke. I immediately gave up the nightshades, the obvious forms, and the pains have really subsided, 100% most of the time but I think I am still getting bits of the nightshades hidden somewhere. For example, I ate some Mexican food in May and it did not occur to me at the time that the sauces on the Mexican food may have pepper in them. About 10 days later I woke up with bad pains in my hip. I seem to have a 7-10 day delayed action, then it passed to other joints — neck, hands, feet, knees, jaws and occasionally the hip. Interesting to me that I do feel a state of euphoria after eating a nightshade, mainly pepper (hot) and the potato. And once I get a nightshade into my system it takes about 2 months to get rid of the pains. My husband is a botany professor so he is very interested in how the nightshades are involved in arthritis. Please send me a copy of your book to help me find the hidden nightshades. SS:Me.

TOOK TWO HANDS TO OPEN DOOR KNOB

I am a consultant on research methods and developments. Six months ago I read an item in Prevention about your work. It suddenly dawned on me that my arthritic problem had started in July as my garden tomatoes began ripening and I had eaten them every day. I also recalled that I had gotten gastro-intestinal distress from eating members of the nightshade family. Potatoes that were not thoroughly cooked gave me violent distress. French fries with uncooked centers gave me problems. Green tomato and pepper relishes gave me terrible intestinal pain not associated with gas. I have stopped eating the four nightshades and discomfort in my hands has left completely. I could not open a door with one hand, took two. I am an R.N. and hope that some doctors will have enough interest in their patients to try this Diet. Almost any drug they use against arthritis or rheumatic pain can do more harm to the body than this Diet. I have severe reactions to even aspirin, so drug therapy is impossible with me. VLVP: Va. R.N.

BOOKS ALL SAY THE SAME THINGS!

About a year ago, I began having pains in my hip and one finger which was swollen. I went to the doctor and he said it was osteoarthritis, take a few aspirins if the pain gets bad enough. I asked if nutrition had anything to do with it, and he said, "Save your money." I then headed for the library to read about this disease. All the authors must have read the same books, as they all said the same things. "Arthritis has been around since prehistoric man, etc., etc." Then I found the Childers' book, bless him! Even though I was not an advanced case, I was determined not to become one. I did not relish the idea that it would take five minutes every morning to get from a sitting position to standing. I followed the Diet for 4 days and, surprise, the pain was totally gone. I have followed the Diet faithfully for over a year now, except when I get a nightshade unexpectedly — the pains last for 3 to 4 days. You are an evangelist. I tell my friends that it costs nothing — all you lose is pain. They think you and I are nuts. I have learned to substitute. My skin rash, since age 7, now 41, I found to be due to milk, dairy products, which I discovered by your suggestion of double-checking when it is bad and not-so-bad, then pinning it down. If you would like to use my case, go ahead. LN:N.J.

SPENDING MY MONEY NOW ON THESE BOOKS FOR FRIENDS

I am 52 yrs and was in a racing car accident 30 yrs ago, when my neck was broken. For the past 2 yrs I have been taking 40 aspirins a day to try to relieve pain developing in my neck, particularly. The medical profession could do little for me except suggest exercises and prescribe pills to kill the pain. A year ago I read about the plan for avoiding the nightshades and asked my wife to cook meals without the four foods. I do not smoke. I improved tremendously, no pain now, but my wife got tired of cooking special meals for me and sent me to a doctor from India to see if he could change me so I could eat the same as she. The doctor told me that they have known for decades in India that tomatoes and peppers are bad for the system. He gave me 6 "neck stretching" treatments and told me to stay with the diet. I would likely have no more problems. I feel young, as I did at 25. I scuba dive, ski, jog, ride a motorcycle most of the time — nothing is a problem anymore. I am so appreciative that I keep spending my money gratefully for these nightshade books and give them to my friends to help them, rather than give my money to doctors and hospitals. ER:N.J.

STAYING ON DIET FOR REST OF MY LIFE!

I have been on your diet for 9 months since I saw you on a Cleveland TV station and intend to follow it for the rest of my life. I had aches and pains all over — ankles, knees, hands, hips, elbows, shoulders and even my toes. I could not exercise due to hurting knees. I was taking all the pain killers suggested for arthritis, off and on by doctor's recommendation. I stopped smoking 10 yrs ago, thank heavens. After two months on the Diet, all pains stopped in my body except my right knee, but now that is gone. I thought Formula 44 for coughs caused me some problem as the aches in the right knee stopped when I stopped that, I haven't felt so good since I was a young girl. I just cannot believe how good I feel, God bless you, after all I heard from the Arthritis Foundation and doctors that little could be done except "grin and bear it". MT:OH.

PROOF ENOUGH

Note: The Courier-News of Somerville, N.J. printed a 5-series set of articles covering the material submitted by the Arthritis Foundation following other articles in other local newspapers about the Nightshades Diet. The articles drew the following letter from a reader, typical of several.

The Courier-News recently published (June 2-6) a series of articles on arthritis by Dr. Fries of California for the Arthritis Foundation.

Nowhere in the articles did I find real help for the arthritic, and the only ways suggested to lessen pain and disfigurement were the use of drugs that have disastrous side effects and exercise, heat; supports, etc. The "help for the arthritic" was just a rehash of publications at least 20 years old.

Dr. Norman F. Childers, horticulturist of Rutgers University, has developed a diet for arthritics after 16 years of research and five years of testing with thousands of "cooperators." His "no-nightshades" diet works. In spite of the recovery of thousands of people (documented) on his diet, the Arthritis Foundation has issued this statement by Dr. Charles Bennett, vice president in charge of public education at national headquarters in Atlanta: "Dr. Childers' book dangles before the arthritis sufferer yet another hope — at best premature, at worst, false." This without any testing or research on the part of the Arthritis Foundation.

I am one of the many people who have had complete recovery from persistent arthritic aches and pains on the Childers' Diet. That is proof enough for me that the "no-nightshades" diet works, if followed rigidly. LVH:N.J.

CAN TYPE NOW: NO FEVER BLISTERS

I continue to improve on the Diet, particularly in my fingers. I now can use a typewriter much as I did when in the business school. Strength has come back to them. It is like a miracle. Sixteen months ago it was very painful to push down each key.

There is another thing you did not mention in your book — fever blisters! Mainly on the lips. I have had them since I was a small child. An ugly sore would appear on my lips then develop into a shining sore like a boil, remaining there for one to three weeks. Sometimes it would almost heel, then start all over again. People became afraid to be near me because of those sores. They often came in my nose which was distressing. Since I have been on the Diet, I am completely free of the blisters. Medical doctors had no idea what caused them and could do little for me. Put this information in your next book if you wish for there are hundreds of people with this problem. WJC:Wash. D.C.

All You Need To

Do Is To Go Back

To The Nightshades

And Your Miseries Will

Be Refunded!

Additional Case Histories

The following case histories were presented in the first edition of this book. They are repeated here in larger type for easier reading, with some up-dating of suggestions.

Mr. JHA; N.M.; 66 yrs; 210 lbs; for 4 yrs; neck, back, hips, fingers; garden, carpenter, nightshades several times/wk; heart pills; spur on heel; diet 10/1/76; by 3/20/77, "Pain, stiffness, lower back gone; finger joints no longer sore; "now I can straighten up after bending over, no pains; so easy to do without these excellent foods when one knows what they do to you. You are conducting one of the greatest programs I have ever heard of and in the right manner, using people instead of animals that cannot tell you how they feel."

Mrs. MKA; Ca; 58 yrs; 138 lbs; for a year; knee, fingers, back; tomato, peppers, quite often; hot pepper; golf, swimming; rash behind ears, over eyelashes; hemorrhoids; diet 8/6/76; by 11/11/76 fingers much improved, writing better; 4/1/77, lower back much better; "if I go off the diet, it sets me back in pains for days. You have helped both my husband and me so very much and we greatly appreciate it."

Mrs. F.J.A.; N.J.; 75 yrs; aches, pains, ankles, knees, back, hands, hips; walking; diet 3/27/76. Almost bedridden before diet, now able to hold balance, walk long periods; pain subsided in neck, ankles, back, hands, hips; left side above knee still problem, 10/7/76.

Mrs. JA; Ill.; 49 yrs; 152 lbs; for 3 yrs; knees, elbows, back; some walking; sinus pills; mostly potatoes, tomatoes; diverticulitis; pain killers; diet 6/1/76; by 11/1/76 much improved, slight pain in knee up steps; "we grow asparagus—it gives me pains in knee and elbows when eat successive days; "slips" always return the pains to me."

Mr. JBA; Ca; 68 yrs; 180 lbs; for 25 yrs; osteoporosis; feet, shoulders, hands; swimming, golf when can; aspirin, Indocin; mostly potato, hot peppers; cortisone sometimes worked; often in Mexico eating hot food; diet 8/6/76; as of 4/1/77 can swim without pain; foot operation in 10/75 still bothers — for osteoporosis; remaining on diet permanently; handwriting much improved; "I think your research approach could improve millions of lives."

Mrs. MLA; N.J.; 32 yrs; rheumatoid arthritis 11 years; in feet, ankles, knees, elbows, shoulders, neck; 14 aspirin daily; doctor destined her to wheel chair eventually; was carried to bathroom and dressed at times; weight lifting, hot baths, showers. Diet 2/3/76, sediment test 29 at start, 19 in fall 1976 and 16 as of 2/8/77; spurs on ankles leaving; toes, fingers, elbows still some crookedness; completely free of pains, but they return with slips on potato and tomato. As of 3/15/77 had sore finger; had operation 1/77; medical advice was relatively high vita. A and D, some E (we suggest lowering or omitting vitamins, for 3-4 mos); overdosing vitamins can cause painful muscles, other problems. As of 5/77 no problems.

Mrs. VGA; N.J.; 52 yrs; 190 lbs; 15 yrs; feet, knees, shoulders; neck, hips; housework; decalgesic helped a lot; mostly potato, some tomato, ketchup; h. hernia; diet 4/15/76, pains subsided some in 2½ mos on diet but pains induced her to go back to decalgesic and drop diet since she thought she should have one or other; as of 5/2/76 going back to diet when found could take pain killers with suggestion to gradually reduce pills with time on diet. Hands becoming swollen, fingers, twisted and 4-5th vertebrae in back affected. Wants to continue teaching piano.

Mrs. VB; N.Y.; 68 yrs.; housewife: aches, and pains 15 yrs: shoulders, knees, hands; aspirin 5 yrs., none now. Exercise: walking, swimming. Diet: 4/7/76; can close hands into fist, swelling subsided by 4/28/76. Neck turns farther, hands grip better, more agile on feet 8/28/76. Husband, 74 yrs., rheumatoid arthritis 15 yrs.: ankles, shoulders, neck, and back, osteo-A for 7 yrs, left foot; under doctor's care; 2 aspirin, 6 Tylenol daily. Exercise; swimming, orchard work. Diet: 3/26/76; within 3 weeks minor arthritic pains less severe in several joints, swimming daily and more agile on feet as of 8/28/76. All pains gone except foot, 5/77.

Mrs. JB; Ill; 71 yrs; 2 yrs; 155 lbs; walking, active all day; Motrin; only few potatoes/wk, overweight problem; back and hips; diet 9/1/76 by 4/7/77 "I am aware that pain in hip is wonderfully improved, finger w/enlarged joint much less painful; quit Motrin; please send more copies of your instructions for friends."

Mr. RB; N.J.; 64 yrs; 168 lbs; tennis, a.m. situps; Motrin; nightshades weekly; diverticulitis; plastic hip; locked ankle; diet 9/1/76; as of 4/2/77 "I have definitely improved staying away from nightshades. After 3 months could see definite improvement, mainly in wrists."

Mrs. RTB; Ill.; 58 yrs; 125 lbs; for 50 yrs; feet, ankles, elbows; shoulders, neck; chiropractor; walking, housework; pain killers, Vitamin C; mostly potatoes and tomatoes; skin rash occ.; citrus may bother sometimes; diet 4/22/76; as of 5/19/76, "general aches have gone, feet do not hurt to walk, noticed great increase in energy and enthusiasm I haven't felt for years. Have cut back on prednisone. God bless you. I don't even miss the eliminated foods. There are so many other foods to take their place and it isn't worth the pain to eat them." As of 5/1/77 no problems except a "tennis elbow" and by phone learned she had been getting bits of potato.

Mr. GC; Ohio; 63 yrs; 210 lbs; for 2 yrs; knee (left bad); right hip, neck; lifting; Motrin, others; all nightshades rather frequently; swelling knee with fluid taken off 3x in 6 mos; diet 4/25/76; as of 11/15/77 "attitude much better, have ambition, feel great, used to be depressed; as of 3/25/77%, today, I feel 100% better than when started, soreness gone from knee, each month brings improvement."

Mrs. GGC; Tex.; 68 yrs; 168 lbs; 1 yr; knees mainly, hips; gardening, housework; motrin, B_1, C, one-a-day vitamins; heart murmur; hard fall on knee started problem; potatoes and heavy on tomato in season; diet 5/1/76; as of 7/76 knees seldom hurt, still taking motrin; "feeling fine — my indigestion, gas, heart burn have greatly improved." As of 5/15/77 "had heart flareup, taking valium, knees sore off and on (had some potatoes recently)." Intends to continue w/diet.

Dr. NC; N.J.; 67 yrs, 225 lbs; problems started 1953 w/diverticulitis (drinking quantities V-8 tomato juice daily); colostomy for 9 mos; stopped tomatoes as caused soreness in ankle, wrist, knee, or other areas after eating them; had 3 breast operations, tender nipples; baked white potato causing pains shooting through ankles, feet in a.m.; stiff knees, hips; tomato causing tingling legs at night, could not get oriented in bed to sleep; stopped potato, peppers (did not eat eggplant), 2/15/75; good health since except when hot pepper creeps into food at restaurants, ache may set in at different place in body at different times, remains for a day or two; no tender nipples; no urination problems; very little aging; liver spots disappearing slowly; mind more alert, do not tire easily, no visits to doctor or dentist in 3 yrs; very good health.

Mrs. ARW; 78 yrs; 145 lbs; ? yrs had problem; aspirin; potatoes, seldom; knees; osteoarthritis and rheumatoid arthritis, high blood pressure; diabetes; neighbor attempting to get her to go on diet for own good; the diet refused and as of 11/10/76. "Probably foolish to stay on mailing list, am not in mood to change all my eating habits now. I try to be careful."

Mrs. NLC; Ohio; 29 yrs; since 22 yrs; knees, skin rash; yoga, housework; nightshades several times/wk; thyroid; diet 10/25/76 found improvement, then eating out had "1000 Isl.Dr., cherry tomatoes, rice pilaf w/peppers, 4 glasses wine, could hardly walk, climb stairs next day, messaged legs to ease aching, tingling, con't 12 days and started 2 days after partaking, had to sleep sitting up on couch for 3 weeks because of pain. "I seem to be very susceptible."

Mrs. DD; N.J.; 56 yrs; 156 lbs; 2 yrs; feet, ankles, hands; bike, calesthenics at home; rather heavy on most nightshades; diverticulitis; diet summer 1976; as of 5/2/77 swollen puffball hands are normal; no deformities; can knit and crochet again; headaches subsided but still get them off & on; eating cooked tomatoes occasionally because were thought less powerful (Suggested avoiding all nightshades in any form, eliminating vitamin pills for 3 mos); "I absolutely cannot touch potato, eggplant and peppers in any form. My fingers swell up and my hands look like puffballs".

Mr. JEC; N.J.; 55 yrs; for 30 yrs 150 lbs; much exercise; nightshades daily; feet, knees, shoulders, fingers, hips, wrists; diet 8/15/76; as of 3/10/77 "I am a spectacular case of quick proof that muscle, bone, joint stiffness can be related to use of nightshades, including tobacco (cigars only 1-5/mo). When I met you in August '76 I was eating voraciously of nightshades from my garden I carefully cultivated and was miserable; beets, spinach and pickles (paprika) affect me; definitely will continue diet."

Mrs. JD; N.J.; 56 yrs; 156 lbs; for 2 yrs; feet, ankles, knees, hands, stomach cramps sometimes; bike, calesthenics; pain killers occ.; mostly potatoes, tomatoes, paprika; diverticulitis, rapid heart occ.; diet spring 1976; as of 10/27/76 - on diet several wks when tried nightshades one by one; potatoes, tomatoes, eggplant and peppers definitely "out" for her. Thinks cooked nightshades have less clout, but eat sparingly when tried; chicken soup and some other canned soups cause problems (they have potato starch in them); nightshades also erupt diverticulitis.

Mrs. JKD, Fla.; 75; 2 yrs, bad knees, difficult to walk and stand w/balance; use walker; dieting to lose wt at 205 lbs; by 4/13/77 diet helped, will stay on it; very little pain in knees now — only when walk.

Mrs. ED; Fla.; 71 yrs; 130 lbs; for 15 yrs; toes, ankles, knees, ears; neck, hips, stomach cramps; bike, swimming; no pills; few potatoes, seasoning; diverticulitis at times; Diet 10/15/76; as of 3/15/77, improved more than realized; over Holidays ate potatoes twice, suffered w/sharp pains on joints, muscle spasms. White wine caused trouble, as did corn chips, Fritos (have paprika on them). "I would be very hesitant to drop diet."

Mrs. RWD; Fla.; 71 yrs; 160 lbs; for 10 yrs; feet, left side and arm, and chest at times as if man standing on it; walking; no pills; smokes occ.; Diet 6/76; as of 9/76 no more chest, arm or foot problems; tried eggplant 9/12/76, got excruciating pains in lower back, could not sit or walk but could lie down; problem gone in 4 days; as of 4/1/77 no problems so long as stay away from nightshades.

Dr. J.D.; M.D., L.I., N.Y., 60 yrs.; Pains, feet, neck, back, 5 yrs.; osteo-A in fingers, one fused; taking aspirin; Exercise; swimming, yoga, whirlpool. Diet: 5/15/76. As of 9/9/76 hands still pain, tender; feet muscles in much less misery; out of bed and on feet easier. After a three-day nightshade intake, felt like somebody had "gone over me with a rubber hose," 2 days later; coming out of it after 2 weeks; Apr 13, '77 — the one finger, no improvement; got green peppers by misleading waitress at restaurant and had return back problem for 3 wks; "If all cooperators who stick to the diet have as much relief as I have had, it is well worth the effort and sacrifice involved."

Mrs. DLD; N.J.; 46 yrs; 270 lbs; for 5 yrs; knees, shoulders, back, neck; vita. C and E; mostly tomatoes, Ketchup; degenerative cervical arthritis diagnosed; diet 11/1/76; as of 3/2/77 neck pains all but eliminated; "I am convinced"; continuing with diet indefinitely.

Mr. LED; Mo.; 67 yrs; 170 lbs; for 3 yrs; feet, neck; mostly potatoes, tomatoes in season, paprika; gout; diverticulitis diagnosed; skin rash; bachelor, cooking own meals; diet 9/76; as of 3/15/77 no dramatic changes in general health; tried tomatoes, potatoes 2x in salad and both times became deathly ill for several hours, followed by headaches for about 12 hrs.

Mrs. RWE; PA.; 56 yrs; 120 lbs; for 10 yrs; feet, ankles, knees, hips; utility in factory; one-a-day vitamin; mostly potatoes, occas. others; in few wks pain in knees gone, ankles took bit longer; no ulcers in mouth while on diet; as of 3/15/77 fine, intend to stay w/diet.

Mrs. AE; N.Y.; 42 yrs; 125 lbs; for 30 yrs; bandage on knees since 12 yrs old; water on knee and drained several times — after fall; diagnosed as lupus and rheumatoid arthritis; destined to wheelchair in mid yrs; blood would not coagulate — warned not to travel or drive for fear of accident, bleed to death; whole body pained, could not lift babies; told problem was inherited as grandparent had severe problem; aspirin and cortisone, chiropractor helped some; diet 5/76; as of 5/1/77 blood normal, no pains or bandage, square and folk dancing; extremely grateful. "Hands, fingers, knee shrunk to normal, ring fell off finger, had to have new wedding ring made. I plan to continue on diet forever. I feel marvelous, haven't felt better in years."

Mr. OVF; PA; 65 yrs; for 11 yrs; 168 lbs; farming, jogging, pain killers; nightshades daily; spinal operation '71 correct sciatic nerve; diet 4/1/76; as of 30 days definite improvement; as of 9/23/76 on diet 100%, no intention leaving it; " I feel very much better, have more ambition, energy, can work longer hours; I haven't had a cold since on diet; as of 3/19/77 diet has done me a lot of real good, awfully glad I heard about it."

Mr. JF; Mo.; 31 yrs; 190 lbs; had 10 yrs; hypersensitive colon, upset stomach; hives occasionally, similar to diverticultis at times; taking tranquilizers, bulk laxative, etc.; week at Mayo Clinic, diagnosed colon not ulcer problem, early 1976; diet 4/10/76; stomach better 6/1/76; settled down to generally good condition by 4/1/77.

Mr. RHF; Pa.; 37 yrs; had 1 yr; 145 lbs; orchard labor; aspirin, butazoladine; nightshades daily, many; osteoarthritis of vertebrae in neck; diet 4/17/76; pain lessened about 5 months later; not been much of problem since (to 3/25/77). Continuing diet.

Mrs. GF; N.J.; 62 yrs; 130 lbs; for 20 yrs; gardening, housework; aspirin; potato, tomato, pepper daily; right hand bad; back, elbows, shoulder; diet 3/16/76; as of 4/20/77 no improvement first several months; the ninth month swelling in fingers went down, left hand wrinkled but normal size; some pain still in right hand, no pain in left, or other areas body.

Mr. S.F.; N.J.; 50 yrs; aches, pains 10 yrs; neck, back; aspirin; diet 5/11/76; aches, pains subsided completely by 10/27/76; playing tennis without pain; plans "to stay on diet until I die of something else"; 3/19/77 "Absolutely, positively, the diet worked; got some spare ribs w/tomato sauce, pains returned in hands and back. I'm strict w/diet."

Mrs. AWG; N.J.; 57 yrs; 110 lbs; for 12 yrs; feet, ankles, knees, hands, elbows, shoulders, neck; wrists; aspirin; unable to exercise much; moderately heavy on nightshades; skin rash sometimes; gold injection; diet 4/2/76; 9/9/76 not sure of improvement "but chocolate hurts me;" as of 3/17/77 "the diet is of help. If I eat tomatoes, potatoes, the pains increase. I think for me it is important to eliminate chocolate."

Mr. LGG; Tex.; 10 yrs; knees, back, wrists; 81 yrs; 120 lbs; gardening, pain killers; nightshades several times/wk; angina; "Yes, diet definitely helped my arthritis in wrists, knees. Was not bad to give up white potatoes after finding what they were doing to me."

Mrs. C.G.; 64 yrs; for 2 yrs; shoulders, back; heat pad; diet 12/1/76; as of 3/15/77 less pain, no heat pad; try tomatoes, potatoes and even chocolate; coconut, some "spices" get aches within few hours.

Mr. EMG; 70 yrs; 144 lbs; for 2 yrs; gardening, "retirement duties", few pills, one for duodonal ulcer; mostly potatoes and tomatoes; painful to take clothes off, raise arm, tingling feeling; diet 5/3/76; as of 8/76 — in 3 wks noticeably reduced pain; in 6 wks 80% reduction in pain; and in 8 weeks, 90% recovery; as of 3/15/77 complete "cure" holding. "I believe you are heading for a Nobel Prize in medicine!"

Mrs. JG; N.J.; for 20 yrs; 43 yrs age; 150 lbs; Yoga daily; aspirin; nightshades several x/wk; no joint disfigurations by x-ray; Italian; many vitamins, health pills; diet 5/1/76; as of 10/3/76 "Pain in hands, wrists gone; feet much better, still some discomfort; hip pain almost gone, neck pain is gone." 3/15/77 Mid-winter had some muscle pains that left by late January 1977; was under tension.

Mrs. CLG; N.J.; 72 yrs; 122 lbs; household work; pain killers; feet, back; nightshades daily; leg muscles bother nights, evenings, diet; 3/30/76; as of 4/10/77; "I am greatly improved by the diet; just returned from Florida where climate may have helped too."

Mr. C.G.,Ohio; 63 yrs; aches, pains 2 yrs; knees, neck, right hip; pain killers; diet 4/30/76; swelling in knees, stiffness gone, pain subsided most joints, knees still slightly sore, 11/15/76; "attitude better, ambitious, feel great, was depressed. Will stay with this one"!

Mrs. CHH; Va.; 56 yrs; 158 lbs; had 16 yrs; feet, knees, elbows, shoulders, breast, neck, back, hips; golf, walking, housework; pain killers; nightshades several times/wk; diarrhea for 9 mos; had allergy problems, took pills; some moles, warts; spur on shoulder and 4th, 5th vertebrae doctor says osteoarthritis; had traction therapy; sinusitis since 1940; hosptialized w/back and muscle spasms; had to cease troublesome medication; hands swollen; hate to go to bed so miserable; diet 11/15/76; by 4/1/77, "I'm markedly improved, but wine or cocktails cause hand hurts for few days; spur in shoulder doesn't hurt; sinusitis clearing up. Best wishes on book!"

Mr. GEH; N.J.; 68 yrs; 148 lbs; for 4 yrs; feet, ankles, knees back; farmer; mostly potato and tomato; skin discoloration, vericose veins; diet 5/76; as of 5/77 all problems gone except some soreness in knees at times; eating asparagus daily increased knee soreness; "asparagus is my favorite vegetable."

Mr. JH; Mich.; 72 yrs; 199 lbs; for 2 yrs; ankles, wrists, stomach cramps; yoga; no pills; nightshades several times/wk; diverticulitis; digestive problems; heart leakage, murmur; high blood pressure; diet 7/15/76; by 10/20/76, swelling left ankle and foot almost gone; slipped on pepper — pains next day; wrist where slammed car door still sore; 3/15/77, "diet did indeed help, no swelling on ankles, reduced soreness of gums; generally feel much better."

Mr. KDH; Ohio; 70 yrs; 160 lbs; for 18 yrs; almost all joints a problem; walking; pain killers plus vitamins; pain severe, some frozen joints; about average eating nightshades; diet 4/1/76; as of 4/77, "I have very little pain any more, and when I eat one of the nightshades, pains return and I quit. Swellings are down and I use no canes where heretofore I used two canes. I think there is something to your diet as my experience has proven this. I do think vitamins are essential with the diet."

Mrs. DLH; N.J.; 68 yrs; 145 lbs; 5 yrs; feet, ankles, knees, elbows; chest (breathing); Bufferin; mostly potatoes, peppers, skin rash, heart skip, small blockage; valium, pain killers; anemia; diet, 6/16/76; as of 3/15/77, "I can manage much better at home, get out and walk at better pace, don't get out-of-breath as did; don't have to stop and rest as often; muscle spasms less; sleeping better. It is very encouraging to me; so happy I attended your lecture."

Mrs. APH; N.J.; 65 yrs; 120 lbs; for 20 yrs; knees, wrist, fingers; pelvic cramps; bursitis attacks; walking 3 mi/day; nightshades lightly daily; few moles; skin discolorations; diet summer 1975; all problems gone in 3 mos; tried nightshades for 10 days, got all problems back, took 3 wks to gt rid of them; "by winter 76-77 had soreness in feet and wrist again, went on Vitamin C, now they are gone and finger joint swelling almost gone, fingers appear normal. Wrist broken 3 yrs ago, arthritis settled there. Pelvic pains and unsettled situation kept me awake some nights for over 25 years. Now in top shape, intend to stay with diet. I think the diet, is *one of most significant, findings in human health in our time.* I believe it is a factor in slowing the aging process, extending healthful life."

Mr. BJ; N.J.; 74 yrs; 148 lbs; for 15 yrs; knees, back; walking, golf; pain killers; liver spots, tumors, moles; diet 10/17/76, in 3 months no problems; as of 3/15/77 "been feeling fine, no problems, continuing diet indefinitely."

Mr. W. J.; N.J.; 65 yrs; arthritis 6 mos; ankles, knees, neck; walking, house work; diet 3/29/76; ankles, knees flexible, cane no longer required as of 10/27/76; eating nightshades caused regression.

Mr. & Mrs. WLJ; Utah; 70 yrs; about 160 lbs; for 5 yrs plus; hands, wrists, back, hips; little exercise; pain killers; nightshade several times/wk; heart problem; diet 5/1/76; by 8/76 continuing to improve; as of 3/15/77 "My wife and I have not eaten nightshades for a yr, both feel much better; pains all left, not about to return to eating nightshades again. We feel you have discovered something very much worthwhile."

Mrs. CJ; N.J.; 52 yrs; office work, aches, pains for many yrs., shoulders, neck, wrists, back, knees; no medication. Exercise: none. Diet: 2/26/76 Pains in knees, neck subsided by 3/29/76 all disappeared by 6/76; Mother in 80s also much improved. Happy w/results. Pains recurred when *Solanaceous* crops tried again.

4/16/77 remarkable recovery, in fine health; mother of 87 yrs now admits potato causes pain; on diet, is not necessary now for her to rub legs with alcohol to relieve discomfort.

Mrs. SAK; Ill.; 60 yrs; 150 lbs; for 5 yrs; knees, elbows, shoulder, chest, back, left hand; chiropractor; walking, rope exercise; pain killer pills; fairly light on nightshades; salt-free diet; an RN; some spine disc damage; about 1/3 of 40 patients in her hospital are problems w/back and cervical pains; diet 8/25/76; as of 3/15/77: "I'd like to say the no-nightshades diet is beneficial. I haven't been completely faithful but I notice when I do eat them, I have more aches and pains". "My mother has a painful and swollen knee and I think she would benefit from the diet but she is 79 and loves her sausage for breakfast."

Mr. HCL; Ohio; 60 yrs; 145 lbs; had 1 yr; elbows, shoulders, hips; mail carrier; walk 12 mi/day; nightshades almost every day; several fatty tumors; hate to give up beautiful backyard garden nightshades; diet 8/10/76; most problems gone by 10/25/76; by 3/15/77, "I am completely free from arthritic problems and intend to stay that way. Here is $10 for the cheapest dietary advice I ever hope to get — intend to abstain from nightshades as long as I live."

Miss ML; N.J.; 21 yrs; 130 lbs; for 9 yrs; knees; hands, elbows, walking; very heavy on white potatoes, all forms; pizza, snacks (paprika), liked peppers; gave up smoking; gave up doctors and drugs — little help, side effects bad; no health problems otherwise; destined for wheelchair; diet 12/1/76; as of 4/27/77 greatly improved, no longer pain in hands that "made me want to cut off my hands"; still occasional stiffness, "but nothing like before"; occasional pain in knees, "first area affected and was in worst shape. I am very pleased with results of the diet". Suggest to her: You are one of the most sensitive to nightshades. Hence, be very watchful of intrusion of paprika in snacks, peanuts, cold meats, soups, check all labels for potato, tomato, pepper products.

Mrs. LRM; Fla.; 72 yrs; 135 lbs; for 15 yrs; feet, knees, shoulder, neck, back, hips; house work, walks; pain killers daily; mostly potatoes and tomatoes; high blood pressure, skin rashes; arthritis worse each year; diet 5/1/76; by 5/20/76 could close fist first time in long time; knee swelling down so can see cap; have energy, ambition now to go places, decorate house; by 4/20/77 still some aches in left shoulder, hip, right knee (one baked potato/mo. eating out); (we suggested omitting *all* nightshades); said should have been on program long ago.

Mr. RM; Va.; 66 yrs; 200 lbs; 8 yrs; feet, ankles, knees, elbows, shoulders, chest, neck; back, hips, aspirin, farm work, heavy on tomato and potato, some peppers; quit smoking 1963; diet 2/15/76; as of 8/30/76, most of pains, aches subsided; as of 5/2/77 had gone back to some stewed tomatoes and was getting pains back in arms and feet.

Mrs. TAM; N.J.; 70 yrs; 121 lbs; for 10 yrs; knees, back, hips, chest; housework, shopping; valium, pain killers; tomato juice often, others little; shoulder spasms; X-ray shows unstable low back; diet 6/15/76; by 3/14/77 had much better winter than last one; still bit stiff on arising, getting out of chair; otherwise fine.

Mr. CM, N.J.; 60 yrs; for 10 yrs; golf, walking; 145 lbs; nightshades daily; diet 3/29/76. As of 3/15/77 — Pain-free elbows, knees, feet, neck much improved; golf 3x wkly; walking; "spreading your gospel to North Carolinians every chance I get. Continue w/your good work. Moved to N.C. early '77."

Mrs. RMN; 47 yrs; 109 lbs; for 2 yr; walking; knees, elbows, shoulders, chest, neck, back; nightshades not very often; mastectomy 1973; tumors on uterus; heavy bleeding at times (rectal); diet 4/1/76; as of 3/15/77 "I have found that tomato, wine, roasted nuts; potato, and "spices" give me pains when I try them. Staying away from these has brought me almost complete relief."

2/15/75; good health since except when hot pepper creeps into food at restaurants, ache may set in at different place in body at different times, remains for a day or two; no tender nipples; no urination problems; very little aging; liver spots disappearing slowly; mind more alert, do not tire easily, no visits to doctor or dentist in 3 yrs; very good health.

Mrs. EBN; N.J.; 50 yrs; 125 lbs; for 2 yrs; hands, knees, ankles, hips; mostly potato and tomato; no pills; diet 4/15/76; had few tomatoes summer '76 — pains in knees; as of 4/15/76 pain almost completely gone, some swelling.

Mr. KFN; N.J.; 58 yrs; 150 lbs; for 2 yrs; golf, on feet in store; tomatoes often, others occas.; pack cigarettes/day; ankles, knees; diet 4/16/76; 3/77 free of problems; tried nightshades twice, got kickbacks.

Mrs. EN; N.J.; 50 yrs; teacher; pains 2 yrs; feet ankles, knees, hips; pain killers; diet 4/12/76; pains had subsided almost completely by 10/25/76; pain in knees returned after eating tomatoes; all swelling down, 12/76.

Mr. & Mrs. LN; Barbados, BWI; 67 & 60 yrs; medium weight; knees, hands, hips; diet 4/76 gave up only tomato, always eat rice or yams, can't eat peppers or eggplant; by 2/17/77, "feel wonderful, entirely free of arthritic aches and pains."

Mrs. JCN; N.J.; 60 yrs; 154 lbs; for 5 yrs; walking, golf, back exercises; tomato, eggplant often, paprika occasionally; indigestion and skin rash occasionally; diet 4/16/76, by 11/5/76 feel better generally, much less pain and aches; tried nightshades, got pains back, twice; thought artificial sweetener causing a problem; by 3/77 free of aches and pains.

Mrs. EO; N.J.; 57 yrs; 140 lbs; for 15 yrs; chest, neck, back, hips; estrogen, thyroid; pills; diet 2/15/76; as of 4/22/77 generally feel good, get around with little or no trouble now; do get aches in hips and knee occasionally; remaining on diet; suggested 2 doz names other cooperators.

Mrs. DO; N.J.; 64 yrs, for 7 yrs; 168 lbs; Motrin; some nightshades often; knees (total replacement); neck,back, elbows shoulders; both wrists; fingers badly arthritic; much arthritic surgery; diet 7/76 to 1/77, "found tremendous improvement, did not resort to Motrin; 3/15/77 then I started to smoke (4 or 5 cig/day), began indulging in tomatoes which proved a disaster; everything flared, mainly wrists, swelling, severe pain; excruciating pain, back to Motrin; back to diet for 2 wks now and results unbelievable; continuing diet indefinitely (stopped smoking).

Mrs. ESP; Cal.; 57 yrs; 135 lbs; for 5 yrs; shoulders, back, hands, stomach cramps; aspirin; nightshades all through cooking, including eggplant every week; gardening housework, walking; diet, 4/15/76; by 10/5/76 back still problem but do feel better, more vim; by 3/25/77 from 8 to 2 aspirin/day, sometimes none; lower back area better, can sleep with no waking pains and decidedly better during day; hands still bit of problem; drank bloody Mary on party, back pains returned, took 2 wks to get rid of.

Mrs. HP; N.J.; 62 yrs; 134 lbs; for 7 years neck, disc damage; Excedrin 10/day; in bed with headaches frequently for 2 to 3 days; diet 4/21/76; stiff neck in a.m. on arising — one aspirin; stiff again late afternoons — another aspirin; "been wanting to tell you what a great job the diet has done for me. I used to have terrible headaches, incapacitating". Tried potato baked, spaghetti with tomato sauce, French fries, separately different days, got "kickback" each time lasting for 3-4 days. Mr. EP; 60 yrs; has deformed hip needing operation, hurts him, diet may have helped some; noticed kickback when he also ate above. Plans operation soon.

Mr. JP; N.J.; 59 yrs; 142 lbs; for few years; sore finger joints; diet 3/20/76; as of 4/1/77, soreness has disappeared; moles fading in color, disappearing; liver spots fading, "My wife and I plan to continue diet to avoid possible future arthritic problems."

Mr. GHR; N.J.; 71 yrs; 135 lbs; for yr; ankles, neck, back, elbows, hips, stomach cramps; golf, bowling; chirop.; valium for ulcer; nightshades several times/wk; peptic ulcer 10 yrs; fatty tumors; diet 6/16/76; as of 3/15/77, "Took 3 mos for all pains to disappear, except neck where injured 50 yrs ago in football — but neck much improved; after 3 mos, tried potatoes and tomatoes and got hip, elbow pains back."

Mrs. IR; Va.; 59 yrs; 155 lbs; for 5 yrs; elbows, shoulders, neck, back; 8 pain killer pills/day; mostly tomatoes, peppers, some potatoes; itchy skin; use of traction for neck; meprobamate with acute attack; try not to get frustrated; elem. sch. supv.; diet 2/76; as of 7/76 freed of aches and pains; trying nightshades one by one found each brought back problems; had more agility and endurance in walking. As of 5/1/77 had pains returning in shoulders and neck, was going back to arthritis specialist.

Miss GR; Mo.; 68 yrs; 138 lbs; for 10 yrs; feet, ankles, knees, elbows, neck, back, hips; mainly potatoes; itchy skin; heart problem due to stress; few moles; one cortisone, no pills taken; gardening, keep active; arthritis all over body now, progressed over ten yrs; diet 7/76; as of 4/1/77 feel more alert, a desire to get things done; body more flexible; pain gone from hands, knees, arm, hips; curvature spine center back still problem; doctor's X-ray knee shows no arthritis now. "In October was surprised to suddenly realize many of pains had gone. I am very glad I started this program and definitely will continue it."

Mr. GMR; N.J.; 22 yrs; 175 lbs; for 2 yrs; college student; aches, pains, wrists, knees; tender nipples, bleeding at anus, anemic; diet 3/76; problems quickly go away on diet; return when start eating Italian foods again; abstaining now (4/15/77), no problems. Mr. JD; N.J.; 21 yrs; also student, college; same problems; in hospital once; diet 1/15/77; no problems since.

Mr. DBR; Nev.; 78 yrs; 135 lbs; for 2-3 yrs; walking, yard work; emphysema, pills; smoked 50 yrs, quit cigarettes 6 yrs ago; nightshades daily; pain killers caused hives; diet 7/1/76; as of 3/11/77, "Now I'm 79 and my arthritic pains have about disappeared — no longer a problem, but emphysema about to get me down."

Mr. JGS, N.J.; 71 yrs; 165 lbs; only potatoes for past several yrs; many pills; diet 4/1/76; No potatoes results in loss of all pains, mainly in back by 4/13/77. Wife also much improved; both continue on diet.

Mrs. C.S.; N.J.; 53 yrs., Sec'y: Aches, pains for 30 yrs., knees, shoulders, elbows, chest and back; arthritis 6 yrs in breastbone, left elbow; was using back-brace, medicinal rub, taking aspirin; under doctor's care. Exercise: swimming and exercising of elbow but pain had increased. Diet: 4/7/76. All pain and swelling disappeared as of 8/25/76; nodes on finger joints gradually disappearing, in good health, no need for doctor; 4/77 feeling fine, looking good, submitting many friend's names as cooperators.

Mr. A.S.; N.J.; 55 yrs.: Aches, pains 10 yrs in elbows, neck, shoulders, back; no medication; osteopath. Exercise: swimming. Diet: 2/13/76. Improvement in shoulder and arm 3/13/76. Pains completely gone by 5/12/76. Golfing, basketball, swimming — no problems, except on eating many sweet cherries, successive days, caused pains in leg for few days; 4/77 completely normal, "stick with diet from here on".

Mrs. M.S.; N.J.; Secy.; 56 yrs.: Chronic arthritis 2 yrs., ankles, knees, elbows, shoulders, neck, back; heavy mental depression; eating potatoes voraciously for potassium content; no medication due to anticoagulants. Exercise: none. Diet: 1/19/76. Complete disappearance of depression, aches, pains in 3 mos., except in right thumb where bone had been removed; thumb tender to touch; almost gone by 8/1/76. Had planned to retire because unable to type, heavily depressed; now quite active; 4/15/77 completely normal, happy.

Mrs. WS; N.J.; 53 yrs; 153 lbs; for 6 yrs; walking, bike; gardening; valium occasionally; mostly potatoes, occasionally others; warts, skin itching, tumor removed; aspirin, supportive shoes; swollen fingers, feet, ankles, back, hips, stomach cramps; diet 12/2/76; as of 3/15/77 helping a lot, much better winter; slipped on few French fries, sore, inflamed thumb, finger 2 days later, extremely sensitive; found potato flour used in doughnuts.

Mrs. WLS; N.J.; 63 yrs; 121 lbs; for 10 yrs; ankles, knees, neck, back; walking, bending exercise; some aspirin; diet 3/24/76; as of 10/76, allergies all cleared; arthritis in knees, ankles general improvement; spaghetti causes ankles to flare up next day.

Mrs. AS; 71 yrs; 10 yrs; 192 lbs; feet, ankles, knees, shoulders, neck; hips; had mild stroke; pain killers; few potatoes wkly; diverticulitis; diet 11/3/76 — as of 3/12/77 "knee pains completely disappeared; hands, fingers without pain, wrists slightly swollen still and angled but pain no longer there — husband can hold my hands without inflicting pain; pain still goes from shoulders to hips to instep of feet; continuing diet".

Mr. COT; Pa.; 56 yrs; 200 lbs; for 2 yrs; knees, elbow bad, high blood pressure; Indocin; diet 3/1/76; pains gone in 6 wks; been partaking nightshades lightly after 3 mos diet, no problem any more as of 3/15/77. Suggestion; this may work for very few people but most people w/arthritic pains can get rid of them only by *complete abstinence* from nightshades.

Mr. PHT; Calif.; 75 yrs; 170 lbs; for 10 yrs; neck, back, fingers, shoulders, legs are bowing; much exercise; aspirin, vitamin pills; diet 8/1/76; as of 3/15/77, "hands, fingers, improved, less soreness and can play better golf, was over 100, now low 90s, hoping for under 90 next 3 months."

Mrs. L.T.; Ore; 67 yrs; aches, pains 10 yrs; feet, back, hands; pain killers; housework; diet 4/5/76; hands greatly improved, pains subsided; sleeping peacefully 11/15/76; ate potato salad and inflammation returned in hands, heels; happy as of 2/1/77.

Mr. BLT; Calif.; 57 yrs; problem 2 yrs; 153 lbs; walking; aspirin; knees, back, neck, shoulders, hips; nightshades daily; diet 8/10/76; as of 11/25/76, "somewhere between diet, medication, I have a new sense of complete freedom from headaches, fatigue; first time many yrs have sense of calmness self-contained ,self-confident, have ability to start small project, finish it, which has eluded me for years". As of 3/26/77, "much fewer headaches, feel calm, and *think more clearly.*"

Mrs. DV; 57 yrs; Wis.; few yrs; 193 lbs; arthritic exercise prescribed by doctor; pain killers; nightshades almost daily; high blood pressure; diet 4/16/25 "had big serving cole slaw w/peppers in it, extreme pain that night that slowly disappeared next few days; doctor interested because he always thought diet had something to do w/arthritis; I'm sure diet is it, based on my return to nightshades time to time; when I awake a.m. am able to do things immediately on diet, no pain at night, terrific." As of 4/1/77, "been on diet almost yr, arthritis almost completely left me. Best move ever made to join co-op test."

Some General Comments

Based on the mailed replies received, the personal contacts and the research background given in this book, the following comments are made. They are tentative and may be changed or further emphasized at a later date. Perhaps you will identify with some of the situations and can proceed accordingly.

Again, if you wish to help with the survey test, we would be glad to have you complete and return the questionnaire in the back of this book.

1. As a summary statement, perhaps the best use of this Diet is to help people with the early stages of aches and pains of apparent arthritis and prevent them from eventually becoming crippled and disabled. The Diet, however, has been helping nearly all degrees of arthritic development.

2. The more of the nightshades a person has been using or eating, if susceptible, the more intense the problems and damage.

3. Cooperators who conscientiously avoid all the nightshades in all forms and stay with the Diet for at least 3 months, preferably 6 to 12 months, **nearly always get good results.**

4. Arthritic problems seem to settle first where there has been an injury or surgery, and these are the locations where tenderness is last to leave.

5. Most people would rather solve their arthritic problems by taking a pill or some quick "cure" rather than give up their favorite foods.

6. If a person has debilitating and excruciating aches and pains of arthritis, he will do almost anyting to get rid of them.

7. If it is a choice between *moderate* aches and pains or the food, some people will choose to keep both the food and the aches and pains and take pain pills.

8. Young people and those with a short-term problem usually recover the quickest, whereas those with crippling problems may take a year or so to begin to show benefits on the Diet, since it took more than a few months to develop this condition.

9. Exercise is beneficial with the Diet to get results sooner. Hot baths, massaging, jogging, golf, tennis, lying in the sun, or any practice that encourages good blood circulation helps faster healing.

10. "Middle-age" cooperators who do not have bone or tendon damage have gotten positive results quicker with the Diet. They also may be able to avoid skeletal damage.

11. Strict adherence to the Diet gets quicker results.

12. Cooperators find that the nightshades are the key culprit in their aches and pains and that weather and other factors have little effect. Cold damp weather probably reduces blood circulation in critical areas which could be tied to slower removal of the toxins.

13. Improvement in the aches and pains often is so gradual on the Diet that you may not notice it. Then, all of a sudden you realize the problems are gone or almost gone. Cooperators tend to forget how bad they were, until they go back to eating the nightshades again.

14. Cooperators who have stayed with the Diet faithfully but still have problems often find the nightshades creeping into their foods as potato flour in doughnuts or bread, paprika in bottled roasted peanuts, on corn curls, other snacks, in spices in pickles; in relish for hamburgers, in tomato sauce cooked in the hamburgers, or tomatoes cooked into other vegbetables at restaurants, or in the meat sauce or in salad dressings. Sometimes it takes two or three months to become acquainted with all these sources where one can get bits of the nightshades, yet enough to perpetuate aches and pains. (See Table I, Chapter II.)

15. With many of the cooperators in the New Jersey area whom we see personally, we have noted a sudden happy look of relief on their faces when they find the Diet is taking away their aches and pains without pills. Some had been destined for the wheel chair or for crippling in one form or another.

16. Pains and soreness may appear within an hour or so with some people after eating tomato, e.g., or for others they may occur the next day, or two days later. The intensity and location of the effect seems to be different for different people at different times. Paprika, just bits, can do the same. Paprika with some people may be felt within minutes as a tingling sensation through the chest, then turn into an ache in a joint a few hours later, or even a day or two later.

17. People who have been on the diet for a few months report apparent increased sensitivity to the nightshades if they "fall off" the diet purposely or accidentally. The body may develop a certain amount of resistance to the nightshades when eaten regularly, and that this resistance is lost after being on the Diet.

18. Some crops such as *asparagus, rhubarb* or *beets* eaten several days in succession in season will cause aches and pains. It seems wise to vary vegetables from day to day, also fruits. It also makes the meals more interesting. Excess *chocolate* and *coke* is a problem with many people.

19. There were three cases of cooperators' backs getting "cricks" after eating potatoes while on the Diet. One cooperator on a visit to Scotland, and who almost "had" to eat some potatoes, found her legs suddenly becoming paralyzed, causing her to fall to the steps she was climbing. Could potato alkaloids (solanine) cause a temporary muscle spasm resulting in loss of protection of the skeletal system by the muscles? Could such a spasm be associated with a "charley horse", or perhaps a heart attack?

20. Many cooperators have reported less visits or no visits to the doctor, dentist and hospital while on the Diet.

21. Cooperators with advanced arthritis, disfigured limbs, bone and tendon damage, after going on the Diet, usually find their condition does not worsen, but after 9 mos to a year or so, swellings begin to go down, and they become more agile and slowly improve. We have noted gradual improvements over 6 yrs, the limit of our tests.

22. We have been able to visit several cooperators in the central New Jersey area who have been having a problem getting results with the Diet. Merely visiting them and discussing how better to avoid the nightshades seems nearly always to help them get results. This seems to indicate that many people need personal encouragement to stay with the Diet and not be half-hearted about it.

23. Overuse of stimulants as coffee and alcohol may cause chest pains. Overexercise, colds, influenza, overdosage with certain vitamins as A, C, and D, and possibly foods other than the nightshades may cause aches and pains. We would be glad to hear from you regarding the latter.

24. People who want to become a part of the survey-test, frequently are the ones partaking heavily of the nightshades. They simply love potatoes, tomatoes, peppers and maybe eggplant. Some also smoke. These people, it seems, sooner or later begin to have health problems, some serious.

25. Cooperators often report sleeping better on the Diet, less nervous, bodies and minds more agile, more ambition, get more work done, more getup, less tired at end of day, more stamina, feel "younger".

26. Some popular drugs on the counter have products of the nightshades in them, as belladona, atropine and scopolamine. Scopolamine is found in many sleeping pills. Most nightshades, including tobacco, have a dulling effect on people, some tranquilizing, and a dulling of brain activity. Cooperators have noted a quicker acting brain and more pep generally while on the Diet.

27. Most of you on the Diet may want to go back to eating the nightshades after 3 or 4 months to assure yourselves that you are on the right track. If you eat them for a week or 10 days, it takes at least this long to get rid of the aches and pains, more often 2 to 3 times as long.

28. Cooperators over 50 yrs of age can remember parents and others complaining about their backs, "Ohhhhh, my sacroiliac is kicking up again. I have a crick in my back." Some walked with a crooked spine, slept on a board or laid in bed with excruciating pains. Some thought it due to a lifting strain, others to a certain model car. "Everyone I know drives a 1947 Chevrolet." These problems seem to develop with people eating the nightshades in quantity, usually during the home garden season.

29. Arthritis may strike at any age, but most cooperators started with the problem around the 4th to 6th decade of life, gradually worsening thereafter. We do have many cooperators in their teens and twenties, probably due to heavy consumption of ketchup, French fries, tomatoes and hot pepper.

30. Some cooperators may be overdosing with vitamins, taking 40 to 100 pills a day. The regular one-a-day pills may be too much for some people who are eating regularly and normally. The body was not built to require vitamin pills under most conditions. Vitamin A, C, D and E should be watched for overdosing. B-complex is often given for bone healing, other problems, as skin eruptions, and for heavy drinkers (alcohol). We have received no complaints on B.

31. Several teenagers on the local university campus are reporting typical relief from aches, pains, stiffness, bursitis, headaches, ulcers, bleeding from lower colon, skin rash, tender nipples, chest pains, when they go on the Diet.

32. "Ingredients" labeling on processed foods is a FDA ruling in the USA, but not in many foreign countries. Hence, with some imported foods on USA grocery shelves it is possible to get tomato, potato, hot peper in a product without knowing it — until the aches and pains develop.

33. Almost everyone, in spite of individual resistances, seems to get a certain amount of arthritis as they reach their 70s to 90s. The nightshades appear to be involved in aging, since once people slow down with aches, pains and stiffness, some becoming crippled, senescence begins to set in.

34. Sensitive people eating at restaurants may find that scraping bits of red pepper skin (pimiento) mixed in peas aside and eating the peas will cause aches to develop maybe a day or two later. Apparently enough of the pepper juice is in and around the peas to do the job. Same thing may be true of moving a sliced tomato aside on a salad dish and eating the rest of the salad.

35. The nightshades probably are related to "Tennis elbow" since this diet has corrected the problem with several cooperators. The problem may develop with heavy usage of that arm.

36. When the nightshades are cooked and the water discarded, they seem to have less clout, but for people sensitive to them, there is still plenty of clout.

37. Cooperators who have checked eggplant after being on the Diet find it to have considerable clout. This coincides with historical experiences with eggplant ("The Mad Apple").

38. Tenderness of breast nipples on men, young and old, has disappeared with the diet for some cooperators. Fewer men have this problem than women, but doctors may recommend removal of the glands after age 50 to avoid cancer.

39. Based on cooperators' replies, smokers should perhaps try to make up their minds to "forget" the habit since there are a lot of disadvantages aside from shortening life.

40. Where bone and tendon damage are severe and of long-standing, some cooperators have undergone surgery at doctor's recommendation, then gone on the Diet with hope of holding the situation status quo.

41. Artificial creams, sweetners and instant coffee have caused some cooperators problems in muscle aches, diarrhea and skin eruptions. One cooperator on the diet said her pains left only after she stopped artificial sweetners. Problems also have been reported with asparagus, beets, chocolate, some wines, liquors, particularly when eaten or used daily in quantity. Check also spinach, rhubarb.

42. Older pets often exhibit arthritis by groaning and moaning from tenderness of their hind quarters and feet. This could be due to nightshades (as potato peels) in the table scraps. Nightshades also may be in prepared pet foods.

43. Some cooperators drop the diet when pains do not subside fast enough, and go back to pain killer pills. They should stay with the diet and continue to take pain killers and gradually reduce them as arthritic problems subside. Pain killers only mask worsening symptoms.

44. One cooperator nursing a baby tried tomato ketchup in her food one day and noted her baby crying, apparently with pain or discomfort, all next day.

45. A few cooperators have reported improved libido with the Diet but this could be due to better health.

46. Some cooperators have had a difficult time staying away from the nightshades. They are too enticing! But after several months of being "off and on" the Diet, they eventually prove to themselves it works and that they can enjoy life much more by avoiding the nightshades completely.

47. People using tobacco, and particularly cigarette smokers, will look the other way when they hear tobacco is involved in the Diet. This is how strong nicotine addiction can be. Many would rather continue the habit, eat the nightshade foods and take pills to kill the pain. But if they hurt bad enough, and this is true of non-smokers as well as smokers, they will start the Diet. Some try to cut down the cigarettes and eliminate the foods. This will not give complete relief, but will reduce the discomfort. One problem is that nicotine seems to give the smoker a nonchalant or rather indifferent attitude toward being rigid about the Diet, and it takes rigidity, not a halfway attitude to make the Diet work. Best approach is to stop all nightshades, "cold turkey."

48. It appears that arthritis likely is a symptom of other diseases developing in the body, as hardening of the arteries, circulatory problems, high blood pressure (a kidney problem), diverticulitis, possibly a heart attack or cancer, and others. The nightshades could be responsible for many of the unsolved human diseases today. Few people are said to die of arthritis. It is recorded as a heart attack, cancer, circulatory, stroke, etc. Once on this Diet, cooperators usually go to the doctor or hospital less and less or not at all.

49. The author has told many of his local friends on the Diet that as long as they stay rigidly with the Diet, they should have less fear of cancer or a heart attack and should add years of good life to their career or retirement.

Note: Please read Dr. George Davis' Chapter VI to note the movement of calcium and phosphorous in the body as affected by a Solanum species and also the effects of Vitamin D_3.

Are You

Really

On The

No-Nightshades

Diet?

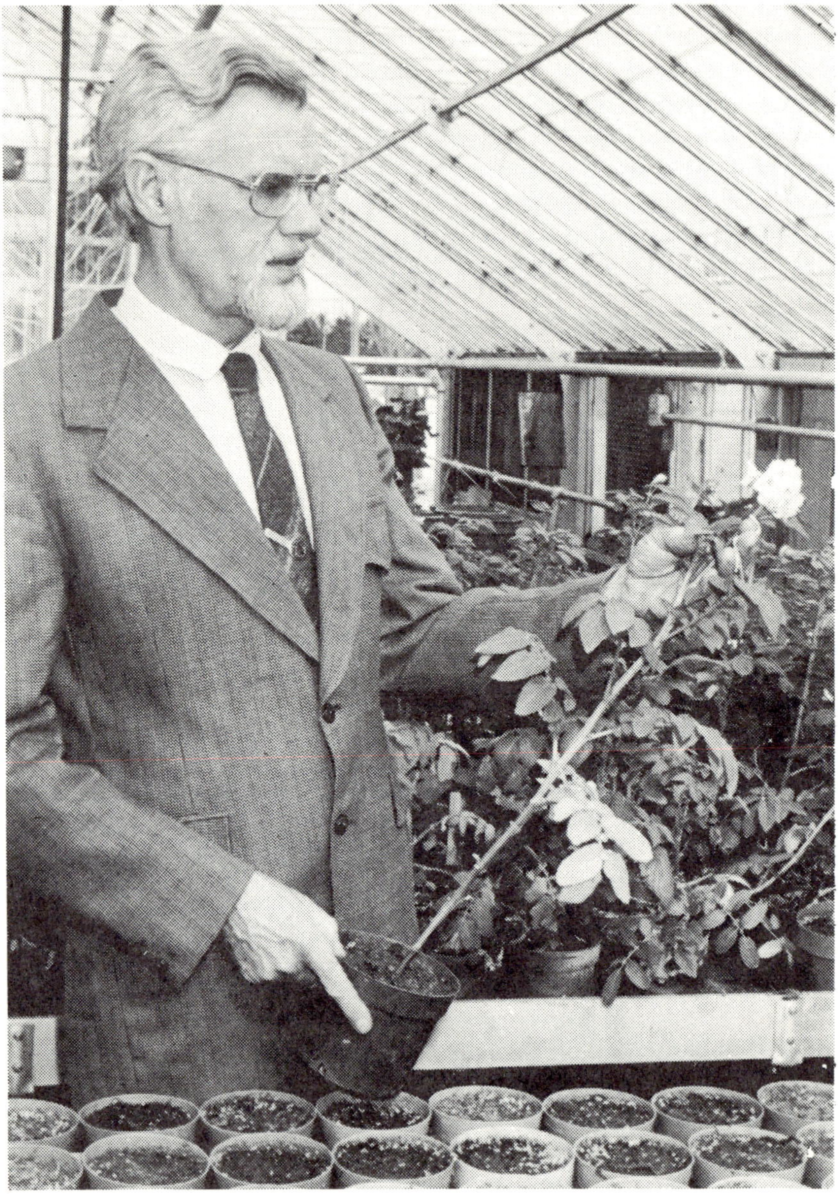

Dr. Ambrose Zitnak attended the Slovak Institute of Technology in Czechoslovakia and the University of Alberta, Canada (PhD). His research has dealt with solanaceous glycoalkaloids, plant growth substances, technology of fruit and vegetable preservation, heat-browning of potato products, physiology of potato tubers, and cynogenetic glucosides. Dr. Zitnak is inspecting B-5141-6 (Lenape) seedling potato, withdrawn from commercial propagation due to high solanine content.

CHAPTER IV

Nightshade Foods — Effects on People and Animals

By A. Zitnak[1]
Associate Professor
Horticultural Science Department,
University of Guelph, Ontario, Canada, NIG 2W1

Abstract — Two types of steroid substances, commonly referred to as solanum glycoalkaloids, occur in solanceous food plants: (a) spirostanols and (b) solanidans. Owing to their striking physiological action based on the steroid nucleus, these substances are of prime concern in human and animal nutrition and in plant breeding involving hybridization of cultivars with wild *Solanum* or *Lycopersicon* species. The abnormal and hazardous levels encountered in edible plant portions are rather rare as these substances, witht he exception of solanines and chaconines almost disappear with advancing maturity. The solanines and chaconines are of greatest health concern as they are normal and persistent constituents of the edible plant part, i.e. the potato tuber, which has an inherent capacity to build-up abnormal levels in response to specific environmental conditions in its post-harvest storage life. Exposure to various light sources, chilling, growth stress and various chemicals are known to induce or retard abnormal synthesis of these toxins, yet we cannot fully explain the sporadic occurrence of 'solanine years' in various geographical regions of the world without further research.

Potatoes with abnormal levels of glycoalkaloids (toxins) possess a bitter, hot and acrid flavor and when consumed in quantity can cause serious illness. From the plant researcher's view it is urgent to investigate not only the total toxin levels and the conditions responsible for their occurrence, but also their individual components along with their physiological action and rate of absorption into the blood stream.

The physiological function and synthesis of the steroids within the plant itself is quite obscure though hinted at by their metabolic rise and decline at various growth phases. Research is essential to resolve the pat-

[1] This Chapter in the first edition of this book was detailed and highly technical, so for the layman's reading, the Chapter has been briefed and somewhat simplified. You are referred to the original Chapter for details of the technical aspects and for references.

terns of genetic inheritance as well as the influences of the growth and post-harvest environment in order to establish remedial measures to prevent or retard undesirable build-up of abnormal levels through the choice of cultivars and suitable post-harvest environment.

The red pepper plant *(Capsicum* spp.) is a singular cultivated solanaceous genus which is fairly free of steroid glycoalkaloids although it does contain in small quantities a steroid glycoside, capsaicidin. With rare exceptions, most of the *Capsicum* species and their cultivated variants produce *capsaicin,* a very pungent, acrid and irritating substance. Capsaicin is the active principle of pungency and spicyness in red peppers and the pungency character is universally appreciated in the use of peppers as a common food condiment. Capsicum preparations also have found wide medicinal application in liniments and ointments because of the powerful and diverse physiological effects of capsaicin. In view of the striking physiological effects of capsaicin and its health implications it was deemed appropriate to include a brief survey of its distribution as well as the current status of pharmacological knowledge.

Introduction

The plant family of *Solanaceae,* next to *Graminae, Leguminosae* and *Rosaceae,* ranks amongst agriculturally important food resources of mankind. Members of this family, the potato in particular, provide staple sources of energy food, minerals and vitamins while others yield raw materials for the manufacture of steroid drugs, tobacco and ornamental plants like petunias, salpiglosis, angel's trumpet, nicandras and others.

The food plants, such as the white potato *(Solanum tuberosum,*L.), tomato *(Lycopersicon esculentum,* Mill.), pepper *(Capsicum frutescens,* L.), eggplant *(Solanum Melongena,* var. *esculentum,* Nees.), Iulo *(Solanum quitoense,*L.) pepino *(Solanum muricatum,* Ait.) and ground cherry *Physalis pubescens,*L) produce a formidable array of secondary organic chemicals and pigments. Some of these compounds represent potential health factors because of their profound physiological effects on animal cells. Fortunately, under normal conditions only negligible amounts of these substances will appear in the mature edible plant parts, e.g. it is well known that the ripe tomato is free of glycoalkaloid tomatine although fair amounts are found in the immature berry and the rest of the plant. It is true, however, that we do not know all the organic chemicals in the food *Solanaceae* that could be harmful to the human body.

From a nutritional viewpoint, the C_{27} steroid saponins and analogous nitrogen containing alkamines are known as flavor and off-flavor consituents, insect and fungal disease resistance factors as well as potential toxicants. the hybridization of cultivars with wild species does often introduce biochemical potentials of synthesizing new substances which may have adverse effects on flavor, nutritional, and health quality. There is a

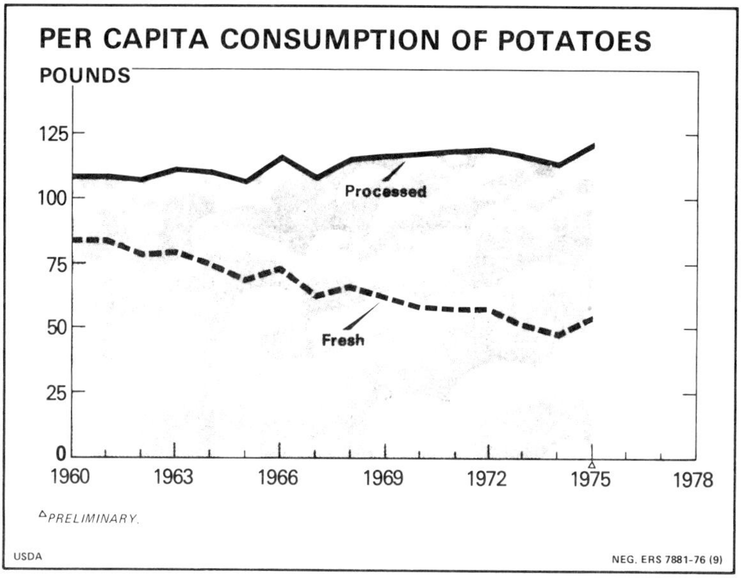

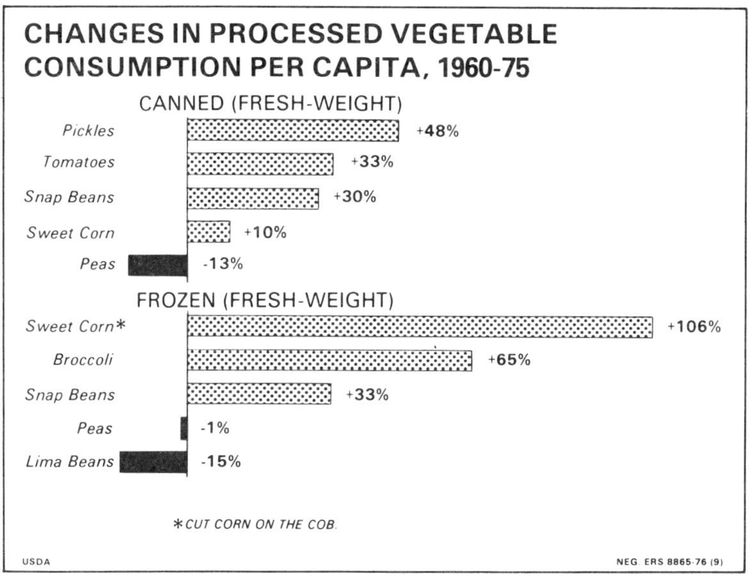

Tomatoes and potatoes are among the biggest food crops in the World. U.S./capita consumption of processed potatoes is increasing as evidenced by over 30 products on supermarket shelves listing them. Per capita consumption of processed tomatoes also is increasing but fresh tomatoes have shown a slight drop. Fast food burger shops move tremendous quantities of French fries and tomato catsup.

tomato line with noticeable bitterness in ripe fruit. More recently, a new potato variety, a hybrid incorporating wild *Solanum chacoense* species had to be withdrawn from production in North America because of abnormal toxic glycoalkaloid content.

The vulnerability of hybrid varieties of the nightshade food plants are of key concern to plant breeders. In addition to the inherent biochemical abilities of hybrids, there is the added vulnerability of individual varities, old or new, to abnormal build-up through synthesis or translocation, of toxic substances in food product in response to injury and to environmental or growth stress conditions stimulating excessive synthesis of these materials.

Thc most common cxprcssion of abnormal build-up of toxic glycoalkaloids is a slow developing peppery, bitter flavor accompanied by a burning perception back of the oral cavity, commonly referred to as "bitterness". The peppery flavor turns distinctly bitter in presence of a weak acid, a common solvent for alkaloidal substances.

The biological activity and physiological effects of these organic chemicals have not been studied extensively and pharmacological information is meagre. The lack of systematic pharmacological information is due to the insufficient amounts of pure substances available for researching. Chronic toxicity studies are non-existent and acute toxicity is still a matter of conjecture although several lethal cases traceable to potato consumption have been reported for humans. More recently, a variety of phenolic and terpenoid compounds have been investigated in the potato regarding possible teratogenic (genetic abnormalities) effects on spina bifida (forked spine) and anencephaly (brainlessness) resulting from eating blighted potatoes.

This review is intended to survey general aspects of the occurrence of glycoalkaloids, their physiological, genetic, and nutritional significance in reference to economic food corps of the *Solanaceae* plant family.

Occurrence of Glycoalkaloids

The first glycoalkaloid, solanine, was discovered by Desfosses as early as 1820 in *Solanum nigrum,* The Black Nightshade, and found six years later by Baup in sprouts of the cultivated potato. It was only a century later that the chemical structure of solanine was described. The companion glycoalkaloid chaconine was found in potatoes in 1954 and in S.[1] *chacoense* in 1955.

The antifungal and antibacterial action of tomato extract has triggered the finding of tomatine, while insect resistance studies have led to the discovery of demissine in S.[1] *demissum* and leptines in S.[1] *chacoense.*

The intensified research since the turn of the century was stimulated by the sporadic recurrence of "solanine years" in which there were incidents of

---

[2] S. denotes *'Solanum'* through the text.

illness and poisoning, the search for insect resistance factors, antifungal and antibacterial agents as well as the search for substances suitable for synthesis of steroid drugs. The search for potential steroid drug resources has been directly responsible for systematic studies of glycoalkaloid patterns in a vast number of wild *Solanum* (potato and eggplant) and *Lycopersicon* (tomato) species and for elucidation of chemical structures of numerous organic chemicals therein.

Thus, from the viewpoint of human health, the glycoalkaloids that occur in the potato tuber or that can be produced therein under adverse environment, should be the prime object of scientific curiosity and concern.

Some Solanaceous Constituents

Tomatine. The distribution of tomatine in various parts of the tomato plant has been studied. The flower parts, immature fruit and plants from which flowering parts are removed showed the highest tomatine concentration while none was detected in the mature fruit. Experiments with tomato scions grafted on tobacco roots showed that the plant tops are the main site of tomatine synthesis and only minute quanities are produced by the roots. The site of degradation is in the inflorescence and maturing fruit while it is absent in the leaves. Old brown and dried leaves were found to have very high tomatine levels.

The tomato seed is free of saponins and hemolyzing substances, however, these are actively synthesized as soon as the young radicle appears; after an 8-day germination period the hydrolysates of young seedlings were found to contain two basic and three neutral saponins, one of the former being identified with tomatidine.

The eggplant, *S. Melongena* is practically alkaloid-free. Eggplants occasionally develop a bitter taste, however, its relationship with glycoalkaloid content has not been investigated probably because of its rare occurrence. It is quite possible that adverse growing conditions or storage environment can induce new glycoalkaloid synthesis similar to that observed in potatoes.

The South-American lulos *(S. quitoense)* and pepinos *(S. muricatum)* are geographically restricted and have not been extensively investigated. The *S. muricatum* steroid aglycone is still unidentified.

Immature berries of *S. dulcamara* possess also a glycoalkaloid degradation system which is activated by ripening. Soladulcidine tetraoside content ranged from 25 to 40% in immature fruit accompanied by solasodine. Immediately before turning red-ripe, the spirostanols are practically completely degraded.

The White Potato Constituents

There are only few detailed studies on the distribution of solanine[1] in

[1] 'Total solanine' or 'total glycoalkaloid' value as based on colorimetric determination of Pfankuch (1937) in which a-solanine is used for reference.

various parts of the white potato plant, while most of the potato glycoalkaloid research to date has been concerned with the potato tuber only.

The highest glycoalkaloid levels are in flowers of potato, no change in the leaf content after 8 weeks of growth, no free solanidine in any part of the plant, and a decrease in shoots, roots and the stem as the plant approaches maturity. Solanidine was previously reported by von Morgenstern (1907) in wilted potato leaves at the end of growth but this is probably due to enzymic degradation in senescent leaves. Wolf and Duggar (1946) have also postulated a destructive metabolism and depletion of solanine toward maturity in the aerial plant portion from initial high levels found in early growth. They have noted that the actual amounts of solanine per plant (hill) increase in leaves and shoots to about mid-season and decrease thereafter; the rates of changes differed greatly with cultivars.

The apparent metabolism of glycoalkaloids toward the end of growth does not follow the pattern in the tomato, where tomatine persists in wilted dry leaves (Sander, 1956).

The findings of Lampitt, *et al.* (1943) were confirmed and extended by Street, *et al.* (1946) by plotting various forms of nitrogen in the growing potato plant. They have reported a drastic fall in glycoalkaloid ('total solanine') in the roots which contained 44-50% of the plant total 8 weeks after planting but only 1.6% 8½ weeks later; concurrently, the plant total for leaves rose from 5½ to 89% while actual leaf concentration decreased from 33 to 14 mg/100g. It is not known whether the root glycoalkaloid is translocated or degraded within the root as growth progresses. The movement into the tuber is unlikely since freshly dug tubers contain 1-3 mg of glycoalkaloid per 100g even in cultivars which have a potential for post-harvest synthesis (Zitnak, 1955). The highest concentration reported for flowers by Street, *et al.* (1946), 618 mg/100g fresh wt., is about 30% higher than values of Lampitt, *et al.* (1943). Potatoes seldom produce berries, and even though three deaths have been cited after berries were eaten by young children (Ruhl, 1951) there are no data available on the amounts or patterns of glycoalkaloid present.

Both solanine and chaconine are concentrated immediately beneath the tuber skin, in the first 10-cell layer of the storage tissue of the potato. Metabolically active tissues such as the tuber eyes and sprouts contain larger amounts of glycoalkaloids than the surrounding tissues. Toward the pith the concentration decreases and the flesh of peeled tubers with normal lev- contain only about 1-2 mg glycoalkaloid per 100 g of fresh weight. Once the glycoalkaloid is formed in excessive amounts, it gradually migrates toward the centre of the tuber. Early after harvest up to 70% of glycoalkaloid can be removed by peeling, whereas in tubers with very high glycoalkaloid content peeling removes as little as 30% of the total amount. In view of these sporadic attempts to determine glycoalkaloid distribution within the tuber, there is a need for a systematic quantitation in various tissues of individual cultivars, with normal or excessive glycoalkaloid levels and over the storage life of tubers in order to assess the effectiveness of peeling in lowering glycoalkaloid content to an acceptable level.

The following paragraphs are presented here to review the aspects of *induced* post-harvest glycoalkaloid synthesis *de novo* since potato tubers produced under normal conditions contain only minute amounts of glycoalkaloids. Numerous researches have shown that the average values for most potato cultivars lie in the 2-15 mg/100g range. The notable exceptions are sun-burned tubers protruding from the soil during growth, a rare high glycoalkaloid content introduced by hybridization and unconfirmed observations on increased levels due to arid hot weather. In this regard, heat-sprouting of tubers occurred in some selections and cultivars in the field due to hot weather.

For many years there was no satisfactory explanation of so-called 'Solanine years' i.e. abnormally high glycoalkaloid (toxic) levels in various geographical regions when portions of the potato crop exceeded the generally accepted safety limit for food purposes. A research group established that cultural practices, soil types and various vine-killing treatments are without marked influence upon toxic levels of tubers while these are attached to the growing plant. Potatoes at the end of growth seem to have normal solanine values. The growing plant, therefore, appears to be able to maintain low toxic glycoalkaloid content in mature tubers within their given genetic potential. This is in agreement with early solanine researches. The abnormal levels are considered due to post-harvest synthesis of toxins and solanine synthesis due to various light sources. The rate of post-harvest glycoalkaloid accumulation is dependent on the variety of potato. Should a sensitive variety receive an induction stimulus within a critical 1-2 week period following harvest, a rapid synthesis of toxins begins within 6 hours and this can continue after removal of the stimulus (e.g. light or field heat).

Such stimulus can be due to injury to tubers (which can be limited to the injured area) but can prevail in mechanically harvested tubers. More effective is the stimulus of harvest exposure to sunlight especially at low temperatures, or various light sources in storage rooms, and on the market shelves.

Numerous chemicals have been evaluated for their potential in preventing induced glycoalkaloid synthesis in the tubers. Systemic pesticides have been found without a drastic effect on glycoalkaloid content of potatoes except a 2-fold increase in greenhouse-grown plants treated with carbofuran. Plants from the greenhouse, however, are known to produce smaller tubers with raised glycoalkaloid levels.

Excessive levels of glycoalkaloids adversely affect potato quality causing a strong off-flavour, a bitter, acrid or hot taste now commonly referred to as potato bitterness. A distinct bitterness indicates near safety-limit concentrations. There are differences in perceptiveness of individuals. Chaconine is much more bitter than solanine.

An attempt has been made to control glycoalkaloid and chlorophyll (green) synthesis by waxing and oil-dips. Several chemicals have been used as field applications and post-harvest treatments. *The current preventive measures to lower responsiveness of potato tubers to induced toxin synthesis must rely on keeping tubers in dark, harvest at high temperatures, minimal exposure to sunlight or artificial light, minimizing tuber injury and using cultivars with tendency for low glycoalkaloid production.*

Another potential measure for maintaining lower glycoalkaloid levels appears to be post-harvest curing of potatoes. Tubers exposed for 10 days to low intensity light after a 10-day curing in a warm dark room (25 °C) showed a nearly 50% inhibition of glycoalkaloid formation. Uncured tubers, chilled immediately after harvest rose from 4.8 to 19.0 mg/100g fresh tissue, whereas cured potato values rose only to 12.2 mg level.

Genetic Vulnerability and Biological Action

The toxins in potato represent a large group of substances capable of marked influence on the physiological activities of animal tissues. *Glycoalkaloids solanine, chaconine and tomatine are bitter and capable of destroying blood cells.* Glycoalkaloids of the cultivated potato and wild *Solanum* species have been shown to inhibit cholinesterase[1] action, and to possess antifungal and antibacterial activity. One of such crosses, seedling B-5141-6, Lenape, was recently introduced as a cultivar and later had to be withdrawn from commercial production because of its excessive glycoalkaloid content inherited from the wild parents. It exemplifies the genetic vulnerability of cuiltivar-wild species hybrids.

Significance for health and Question of Toxicity

Concern about the influence of solanaceous food plants upon human and animal health arises from the steroid components of saponins and glycoalkaloids, which are the source of the powerful physiological action of steroid hormones and drugs. From the consumer viewpoint, some saponins and glycoalkaloids are alleged flavour constituents as they usually occur in amounts insufficient to cause distinct off-flavours, bitterness and acrid or hot flavours. The characteristic potato flavor is attributed to solanine.

The mature tomato fruit is free of tomatine, as the fruit was demonstrated to be the site of tomatine degradation. Likewise tubers of most potato cultivars contain very low amounts of solanine and chaconine. With the exception of certain genetic lines the majority of saponins and glycoalkaloids occur in very low amounts in the edible plant portions. The solanaceous plants are generally more dangerous to animals accidentally feeding on plant tops which often contain considerable amounts of toxins. Withered potato tops fed to goats, sheep and oxen in Cyprus were not

[1] An enzyme in your muscles that affords agility of movement; when inhibited there is stiffened muscle movement.

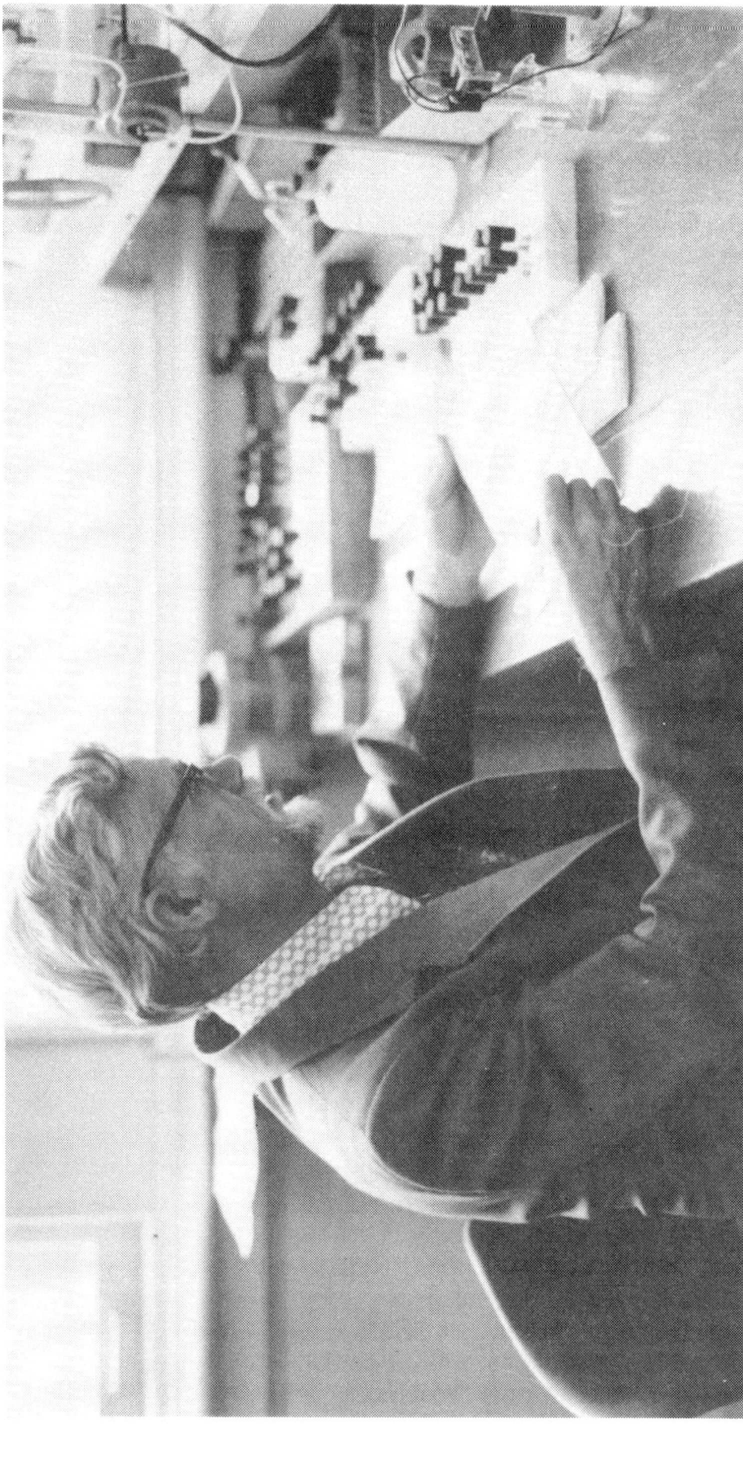

Dr. Ambrose Zitnak has devoted most of is research life studying the chemistry of the nightshade food plants, a world authority. Here, he reviews this manuscript in his laboratory, Department of Horticultural Science, University of Guelph, Guelph, Ontario, Canada. N1G2W1.

harmful, but sickness and death of animals resulted from feeding on unwithered fresh plant tops.

Numerous instances are cited in the literature of poisoning of cattle, pigs, sheep and goats feeding on shoots or suckers of the tomato, on potato vines, peelings, sprouts of sun-burned potatoes, and on plant tops of numerous ornamental or wild species of this large nightshade family is well known although in many cases not supported by feeding experiments with animals.

Most of the reported incidents of poisoning in humans or animals are of acute nature which, if not lethal, are followed by illness of varying severity with recovery within a few days or even hours and no apparent after effects. Fortunately, lethal cases are rare amongst humans, they are more prevalent amongst domestic animals as they feed, often accidentally, on plant tops rich in various glycoalkaloids.

The unripe fruit of the ground-cherry of Hawaii, *Physalis peruviana* (Cape gooseberry) is considered definitely poisonous. Another ground-cherry, *P. longifolia* has been suspected of poisoning sheep. It is possible that berries of the potato, blamed for 3 recorded accidental deaths of children lack the degradative mechanism demonstrated in the maturing tomato fruit. The garden huckleberry, *S. intrusum,* is also likely to have a strong degradative mechanism in the edible berry as it is considered non-toxic. Bittersweet, *S. dulcamara* has also caused losses of cattle, horses and sheep in Europe, and its berries were suspected for poisoning of children in America.

The eggplant is reported practically free of glycoalkaloid and has not been involved in animal poisoning. There is only one previous unconfirmed report on presence of solasodine in bitter eggplant fruit. However, in The American Encyclopedia (1946) is the statement, "'It (the eggplant) was formerly regarded as noxious; in which account Girarde (1597) entreats his countrymen to eschew it."

The author has noted two incidents of bitterness in fruit of the eggplant, *S. melongena,* in one North American cultivar and in one native to Nigeria, both of which gave positive high alkaloid tests, and in the immature berry of the tomato eggplant, *S. integrifolium;* all berries were exceedingly bitter, yet the Nigerian eggplant is a common food source for natives.

Potato "Poisoning." Green berries of potato plants eaten by children and resulting in their deaths have been probably the first incidents which have hinted to the presence of a toxic material in potatoes. A fatal case is reported from Cypress of eating boiled young potato shoots, a custom prevailing at that time amongst inhabitants of mountainous regions. Although the assay of potato sprouts showed relatively low solanine (27.0 to 48.9 mg/100g by gravimetric method) the glycoalkaloid was held responsible for about 50 cases of gastro-intestinal sickness of varying severity including one death.

From the pharmacological viewpoint the anti-cholinesterase effect of potato glycoalkaloids may well be involved in the ill effects of solanine or glycoalkaloid intake. The inhibitory effect of aqueous extracts of various parts of the potato plant has established and was related to solanine content with plasma and erythrocyte cholinesterase inhibitation in rabbits. There are three differential types of inhibition which can be speculated to be the basis of sensitivity of human phenotypes to glycoalkaloid intake. A rapid recovery of serum cholinesterase has been noted without inhibition of red cell cholinesterase after small multiple administration of a-solanine. Since *a-solanine has been shown to produce a depression of the central nervous system and a paralysis after intravenous injection, cholinesterase as a transmitter of nervous impulses may well be affected by glycoalkaloids even though the rate of a-solanine absorption into the blood stream was estimated at only 1%.* The question of course cannot be resolved until further evidence is assembled concerning the pharmacological effects of glycoalkaloid components other than a-solanine and particularly the rate of their passage into the blood stream.

The 'solanine' health problem is of singular importance for the potato tuber, a primary staple food of a large segment of world population with per capita consumption over 50 kg p.a. in North America and in excess of 150 kg p.a. in Eastern Europe. Among solanaceous plants the potato tuber has the unique capacity to trigger post-harvest glycoalkaloid synthesis in response to light induction. Most of the other solanaceous plants are capable of metabolic degradation of glycoalkaloids in the ripening fruit. Yet, in spite of all research, the unequivocal proof of solanine lethality in reported fatalities is still outstanding, considering the large oral dosage (225 to 1000 mg/kg) necessary to produce pathological effects in animals. A case is recorded where an oral 400 mg dose of solanine was taken by a man and described the subequent ill effects and eventual full recovery. There is no doubt that solanine illness or ill effects do occur after ingestion of potatoes with excessive glycoalkaloid content as the author personally encountered several cases of such illness in 1952 and in 1954 in Western and one in Eastern Canada which led to the discovery of high glycoalkaloid levels in the Lenape cultivar. *The main reason for some doubts about solanine toxicity is simply the existence of numerous related compounds,* e.g. the solanine and chaconine series of mono-, di-, and trioses, the occurrence of solamarines and leptines from *S. tuberosum* x *S. chacoense* hybrids. Most of medical and toxicological studies up to date are based on *in vitro* studies of haemolysis, anticholinesterase activity and the injection of solanine intraperitoneally or directly into the blood stream. *Virtually nothing is known about chaconine and its lesser glycosides, although chaconine was reported to represent 60% of the total glycoalkaloid content of the potato tuber.*

Much of the early work on solanine "poisoning," traceable to ingestion of potatoes with high solanine content, is poorly documented or supported through general pathological diagnosis and reliable assays of suspected potato lots. Many of the described occurrences involved large groups of individuals and illness traceable to potatoes with high solanine content. The bacteria toxin theory cannot be totally rejected since cooked potatoes provide an excellent growth medium for microorganisms; recent researchers have shown the capacity of certain organisms to be capable of destruction of steroids and thus modify their chemical and physical behavious, e.g. solubility or absorption rate into the blood stream. The water-solubility of leptines is a most fitting example in this regard. Even if the microbial modification is proven to produce a toxic agent, the original glycoalkaloid must be considered as the primary casual agent of illness.

Poisoning Symptoms. The general symptoms of high solanine ingestion are fairly well described in the literature. The symptoms are listed as moderate to severe gastrointestinal inflammation, nausea, diarrhea, vomiting with large dosages, abdominal convulsions, decreased pulse rate and perspiration, headache, dilation of pupils, throat irritation, weakness, exhaustion and finally partial paralysis and coma.

The 'solanine' health problem cannot be defined in simple terms of chronic and acute toxicity or a definite intake tolerance and toxicity level beyond which human or animal health will be adversely affected. There is an apparent species difference in sensitivity to solanine in animals and probably also amongst humans. People with functional liver disorders are more sensitive to solanine intake. There also is a large variation in taste preception as only 50% of a taste panel were able to detect glycoalkaloids in potatoes in the 10-20 mg/100g range, 75% in excess of 20 mg and 2% were unable to detect any bitterness at a 50 mg/100g level.

Bomer and Mattis (1924) said a solanine content of 20 mg/100g fresh wt. of potatoes as the tolerance limit beyond which potatoes are unfit for consumption; Wilson (1959) gives a 20-25 mg range for toxic effects. These values have been generally cited by most authors for lack of further research. The skin or "jacket" of the potato, and just under it, are higher in solanine content than the inner flesh. There is an urgency to determine oral dosage effects and absorption rates for related toxins known to occur in potato tissues before any definite intake tolerance limits are set. These should take into account the average portion of potatoes included in a meal.

An elaborate hypothesis has recently been presented associating teratogenic birth defects, spina bifida and anencephaly with consumption of blighted potatoes. But one group of researchers were unable to demonstrate clearly these defects in pregnant rats or marmosets fed with a concentrate of blight-infected potatoes. There is no experimental evidence to relate a-solanine, a-chaconine, rishtitin and phytotuberin to anencephaly and spina bifida. Further research is needed on solanine in relation to pregnancy. In a diet containing 10% of potato sprouts and a-solanine fed to pregnant rats only about 50% of the rat pups survived.

Needed Research. *Thus, in order to resolve the question of toxicity, solanine and related glycoalkaloids must receive further attention regarding their influence upon human and animal health, the differences amongst species and individuals as well as the sensitivity relating to pregnancy.*

Editor's Note: As this book goes to press, we received from a doctor cooperator in California the following abstract of an interesting research paper published by M. McMillian and J.C. Thompson in the Qtrly. Journ. of Medicine (England) 48: 227-243. 1979 entitled, "An Outbreak of Suspected Solanine Poisoning in Schoolboys".

Seventy-eight schoolboys became ill after eating potatoes at lunch on the second day of the autumn. Seventeen needed hospital admission, 3 being dangerously ill. Symptoms, which came on 7-19 hours after the meal, included vomiting, diarrhea (sometimes profuse) and generalized abdominal pain, leading in one boy to an appendectomy. Prominent also were a variety of neurological disturbances, including drowsiness and coma, delerium, extreme restlessness, confusion, hallucinations and visual disturbance.

The first clue to the cause of the outbreak came when the affected boys were found to have low levels of plasma cholinesterase activity. Solanidine alkaloids, or potato extracts containing them, are known to depress human plasma cholinesterase activity in vitro. A potato extract from peeled, boiled potatoes left over from the meal was estimated to contain 25-30 mg of solanine/100 g potato; most whole potatoes contain less than 10mg/100g, and most of this is in the peel. The outbreak is thought to have arisen because potatoes left over from the summer term were used in preparing the meal, and high levels of alkaloid had accumulated during storage, possibly as a result of exposure to light.

The authors review the chemistry of solanidine alkaloids and discuss the reasons why solanine poisoning is so uncommon. Partly, it is due to the fact that, since the alkaloid is mainly present in the peel and is also water soluble, most of it is removed by peeling and boiling. Another possibility is that isolated cases are easily overlooked. The true frequency of excess exposure remains unknown and this may have significance in relation to possible teratogenic effects (physical abnormalities).

The Capsaicinoids (Peppers)[1]

The red pepper belonging to the genus *Capsicum* of the *Solanaceae* plant family, in its great variety of wild and cultivated forms, produces *capsaicin* the pungent principle responsible for the hot, peppery flavor of capsicum fruit appreciated as a food condiment and a spice. Capsaicin is

[1]The Eastman Kodak Company, Rochester, N.Y. 14650 has developed a powerful pepper substitute advertised for flavoring, namely 2-iso-Butyl-3-methoxy-pyrazine.

lacking in some sweet pepper cultivars the source of sweet paprika spice savoured and probably originated in Central Europe.

The capsicum pods were and still are a valued item of the spice and drug trade, a staple food item in many tropical and subtropical regions of the world although the importance of capsicum oleoresins, ointments and tinctures are of lesser medicinal use than in the past.

There is a multitude of common regional names given to various forms of the capsicums, such as cayenne, chillies, bell pepper, red cluster pepper, cherry pepper, bird pepper, etc., which are variants of one species, *C. annuum*. This probably is true of the North American cultivars, however, studies indicate the probable existence of 4-5 species. There appear to be three commercially important species, *C. minimum* Roxb, and *C. frutescens* L., tropical plants with small and very pungent fruits commonly known as 'chillies', and *C. annum* L. from which are derived "capsicum", "cayenne pepper" and "paprika". The latter species is a plant of temperate climates with a wide variation of fruit shape, size and color but generally much less pungent than chillies.

In view of the classification difficulties and disagreement of taxonomists, it is not surprising that the plant materials used in capsaicin studies are often inadequately identified in taxonomic terms. Nevertheless, the wide distribution of capsaicin throughout the native and cultivated forms of *Capsicum* is well established and documented. Because of the striking physiological effects of capsaicin on animal cells and tissues and the extensive use of capsicum preparations in medications of the past century, extensive pharmacological information has been accumulated. With the current advances in isolation and improved assay methodology, there appears to exist a renewed interest in reinvestigation of capsaicin of C. resources as well as in awakened pharmacological studies.

There is a need to stimulate further researches concerning the capsaicin distribution and variability in relation to plant growth, environmental factors affecting its synthesis and the post-harvest physiology of the crop as well as its handling in trade channels. This will no doubt create added stimulus for a reappraisal of the capsaicin effects on animal and human physiology and its nutritional and health significance.

The pungency of peppers may be adequately described by the term 'total capsaicinoid content' since it is not known whether individual capsaicinoids can impart pungency of varying intensity or whether they excite differential sensory and physiological responses in human and animal bodies. From the viewpoint of human health the latter should certainly be a matter of common concern of pharmacologists, physiologists and biochemists.

Although a century has elapsed since the discovery of capsaicin, with most of the research interests being focused on its medicinal and pharmacological properties and uses, there is only scanty information on its distribution in the plant, on factors affecting its formation, inheritance, variation during plant growth and its metabolism or synthesis within the plant. With the improvements in capsaicin and capsaicinoid methodology over the past decade, there is indeed an open challenge to plant physiologists, biochemists, and agronomists to assemble reliable data on (a) seasonal fluctuations, on (b) species and plant distribution, on (c) inheritance of the pungent character and on (d) its metabolic transformations within the plant as well as (e) its fate in the animal organism.

The sweet paprika spice is not completely free of capsaicin which is present at 1-3 mg/100 g concentration. Sweet varieties of red pepper contain less than 0.020% of capsaicin on fresh weight basis.

A survey of chemical composition of 15 red pepper varieties from Czechosolvakia, Bulgaria and Hungary disclosed very high levels of ascorbic acid (109-292 mg/100g), capsaicin content below 0.020% in 12 'sweet' and 0.05 - 0.14% in 3 'hot' pepper varities, and only a negligible change in capsaicin in 'sweet' varieties at three stages of maturity. In 'hot' varieties there was a slight increase in capsaicin and a substantial increase in ascorbic acid content.

Capsaicin begins to accumulate about 4 weeks after pollination of blossoms and can be mainly found only in the seed placenta (1.794%) with very little in the seed itself (0.070%) and in the pericarp (0.101%) giving an overall concentration of 0.492% in the whole fruit of *C. frutesens*. Smaller fruit contains usually more capsaicin than larger fruit and the maximum content is reached at the green-mature stage followed by a slight drop during further ripening. Attempts to assess the influence of environmental conditions, soil medium and inheritance of capsaicin, are practically non-existent.

Pharmacology

Capsaicin is a powerful irritant causing a burning pain sensation of skin and mucous membranes and its introduction into an organism has profound physiological effects, such as pain desensitisation, hypothermia, and irritation of circulatory and respiratory receptors. The frequent usage of capsicum in tinctures, liniments, ointments and other early medications is therefore not surprising although their importance has diminished with the advent of modern drugs. As reflected in the increasing number of published papers over the past decade, there is a renewed interest in reevaluation of the physiological effects of capsaicin. Historically, capsicums played an important role in social and religious customs and rituals of primitive people much beyond its use as a culinary spice and a common medication of the past century.

Physiological effects. Capsaicin produces a great variety of physiological responses affecting various body functions, *such as cardiovascular, respiratory, and digestive systems as well as desensitisation against chemical stimuli.* These effects involve the following: (a) strong irritation of circulatory and respiratory reflexes; (b) intensification of gastric peristalsis; (c) stimulation of gastric acid production in small and inhibition in large doses; (d) mild inflammations and burning sensation of skin and mucous membranes; (e) desensitisation of animals to chemical stimuli on prolonged treatment; and, (f) *in toxic doses, capsaicin causes fatal hypothermia and symptoms similar to an anaphylactic shock which could result in collapse or death.* There is o clinical evidence as to the acute toxicity of capsaicin to man probably due to the deterrent of strong irritation excited by intake of highly spiced foods. The long term effects of chronic toxicity or ill effects of a capsaicin containing diet yet are to be determined. The external irritation of skin, eyes, nasal, and bronchial passages by capsaicin is well knwon and is the basis of some animal repellant spray formulas. It is also an ingredient for penetrating bronchial liniments.

In animals a differential sensitivity to capsaicin was noted by several researchers. The lethal dose for anaesthetized cats by infusion was found to be 1.56 - 4.3 mg/kg. It was less toxic to mice and rats and about 20-times weaker in rabbits. *The most sensitive animal is the guinea pig which succumbs to capsaicin induced hypothermia. Parentheral doses of 0.5 mg/kg cause death from a histamin-like and anaphylactic shock resulting in suffocation and spasms of small bronchiae.*

In the past decade the physiological actions of capsaicin have been reinvestigated and reconfirmed by several investigators. One researcher observed an irreversible impairment of body temperature regulation in rats and guinea pigs. Capsaicin-desensitized animals lost protection against over-heating, i.e. responded with hyperthermia at 32-4030C attributed to the impairment of heat dissipating mechanisms rather than to increased heat production.

Capsaicin failed to block sensitivity to pain-inducing chemicals but produced long-lasting insensitivity to irritants applied to mucous membranes. *Capsaicin-stimulated synthesis of prostaglandins is considered a causal factor in headaches and digestive tract disorders.* There is a sensory irritability by capsaicin of the upper respiratory tract in mice followed by desensitisation to sulfur dioxide and other chemicals.

There are indications of a reduced fat absorption in rats placed on 4- and 8-week capsaicin diets. Subsequently, intraduodenal and intragastric administration was shown to damage duodenal cells with apparent deformations in mitochronrdria, nuclei and chromatin. Cardiovascular responses to capsaicin have been studied by Ueno (1971) and Toda, *et al.* (1972) in anesthetized dogs. Fukuda and Fujiwara (1969) have found increased contraction amplitudes of isolated guinea pig atrium and determined that capsaicin action is different from and independent of adrenaline.

Vascular responses to stimulation of pulmonary and carotid baroreceptors by capsaicin have been elucidated by Brender and Webb-

Peploe (1969). An interesting observation has been made on the antibacterial effect of capsaicin; a growth inhibition was exhibited by several microorganisms, the *Bacillus subtilis* and *B. cereus* being most sensitive with a measurable inhibition at 10 mg/ml.

The foregoing brief review of capasicin pharmacology is by no means exhaustive but a good indication of renewed interest on its physiological action. Further current information is now more easily accessible than that of earlier workers.

Note: As this book goes to press, one of our cooperators from North Carolina sent us a clipping from a Richmond, Virginia newspaper telling about a North Carolina State University entomologist working with a colleague plant breeder to develop a tomato hybrid resistant to the main insect enemies of the tomato. This would reduce the need for chemical pesticides. They are using a small-fruited South American tomato with hairs that exude a liquid that kills the pest within 20 minutes on touching it. They are cross-breeding with a large-fruited tomato to get size and quality. The scientists no doubt will consider possible toxicity to humans before introducing an improved hybrid of this nightshade. But this information does indicate the toxicity that some nightshades can develop.

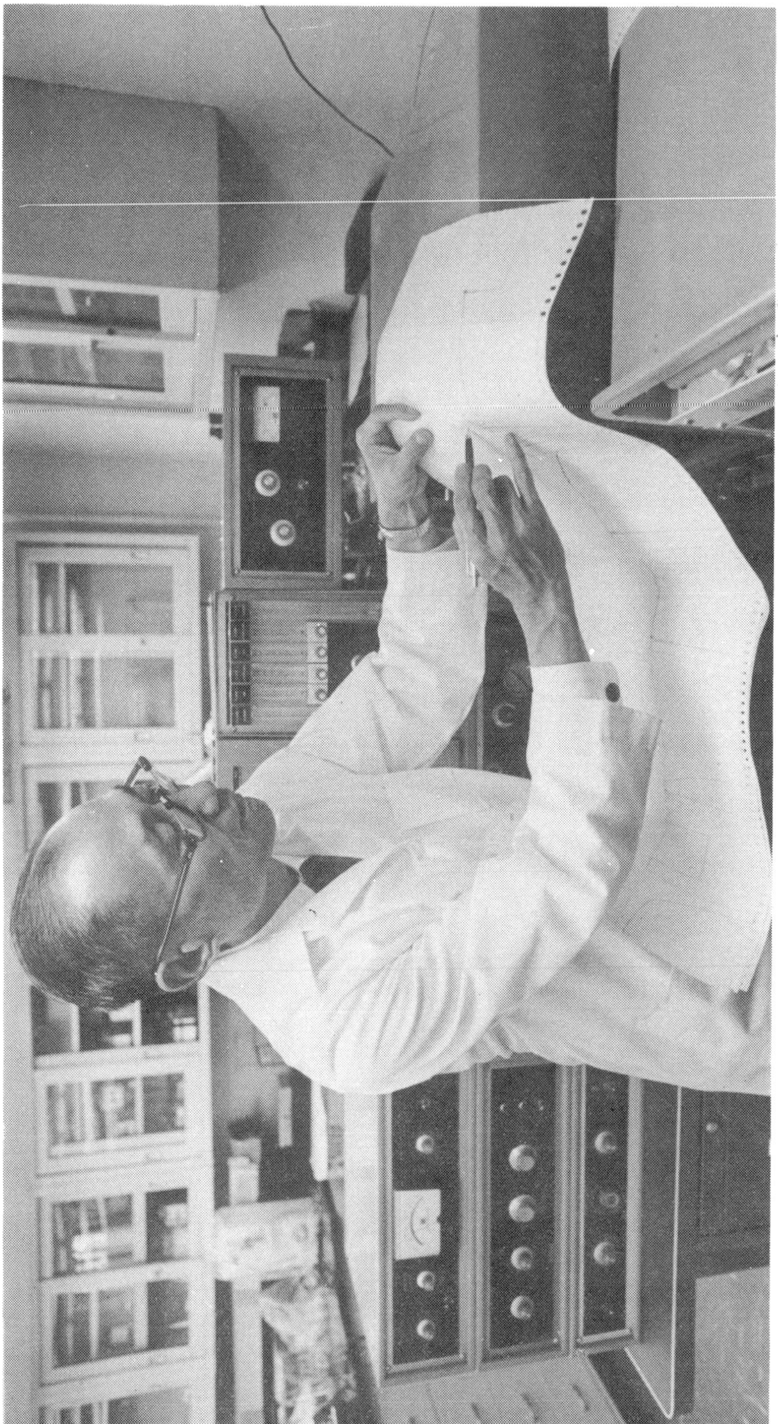

Dr. Tien Chioh Tso received his B.S. and M.S. degrees from Nanking University, China and his PhD from Penn State Univ., 1950. He is a phytomchemist and Leader of the Tobacco Laboratory, U.S. Dept. of Agric., Beltsville, Md. 20705.

CHAPTER V

Tobacco Nightshade and Tobacco Smoke

By T. C. Tso, Chief
Tobacco Laboratory, Beltsville Agricultural
Research Center, Agricultural Research
Service, U.S. Department of Agriculture
Beltsville, Maryland 20705[1]

Introduction

Tobacco *(Nicotiana tabacum L.)* is mainly used for its combustion products which induce physiological effects. There are 4,500-5,000 compounds which have been identified in leaf tobacco and tobacco smoke. Indications are that at least 30,000 additional compounds may be present in tobacco smoke. New compounds are being reported almost every day. Most of these new compounds are, however, in very minute quantity. It would be an impossible task to examine the biological significance of each leaf and smoke component known to us. This chapter will provide general information on problems associated with smoking and health, major tobacco and smoke constituents, and potential beneficial products of tobacco.

The tobacco industry is very conservative and slow to change until the last 10 to 15 years. The rising cost of tobacco production and the health problems associated with tobacco smoking made it necessary for such changes. Much information is available on the current status and future prospects of this important economic crop, its benefits as well as its potential hazard.

Tobacco Production

Tobacco was introduced by John Rolfe from the Indians of Eastern North America for cultivation in Virginia in 1611. It was introduced into Europe in the middle of the 16th century and to Asia and South Africa early in the 17th Century. Tobacco is now being produced and marketed in most parts of the world.

Trend of world production. World tobacco production was on the increase in the early 1970's, but has gradually stabilized in recent years. For example, during the years 1975, 1976, and 1977 the total volume of tobacco harvested was 4.34, 4.36, and 4.37 million hectares; yields per

---

[1]Mention of a trademark or proprietary product does not constitute a guarantee or warranty of the product by the U.S. Department of Agriculture and does not imply its approval to the exclusion of other products that may also be suitable.

In this second book edition, much of the technical data and references have been omitted. Please see the first edition for these omissions.

hectare were 1211, 1277, and 1243 kilograms and total production was 5.37, 5.57, and 5.43 billion metric tons.

Asian countries lead the world in tobacco production, followed by North America, Europe, and South America in decreasing order. The yields per hectare were lowest in Africa, followed by Asia, South America, Europe, Oceania, and North America, in increasing order. In 1977, the People's Republic of China produced 975 million metric tons of tobacco; the United States had 874 million metric tons; followed by India, USSR, Brazil, and Turkey in decreasing order.

Based on the 1976 data, the United States led the world in tobacco exports, and United Kingdom and West Germany were first and second in total amount of tobacco imports during that year. U.S. tobacco is well known for its excellent quality and is highly prized for desirable cigarette blending.

U.S. tobacco classification and production. Freshly harvested green tobacco leaf is not used for smoking purposes. The first process to bring about the development of a pleasant taste and aroma of the harvested leaf is "curing". It is carried out by hanging the fresh leaves in barns under regulated conditions of temperature and humidity. Tobacco leaves are either harvested and cured individually when ripe, known as "primed" or "picked" leaves, or the whole plant is cut and cured with leaves remaining attached to the stalk, known as "stalk-cured."

Bright tobacco, also known as flue-cured tobacco, is always primed while most air-cured leaves are stalk cured. Flue-curing takes its name from a system of large pipes or flues that heat the curing barn throughout the curing period of 4-5 days. However, open-flame gas or oil burners are now most widely used for flue-curing. Fire-curing is accomplished by the use of hardwood fires which impart a characteristic odor and taste to the cured leaf. Tobacco cured without the use of artificial heat, except in some cases during periods of wet weather, is called air-cured tobacco. In such cases, the tobacco is placed in the barn and curing is controlled by regulating the ventilation of the building.

Based on different methods of curing, leaf tobaccos produced in the United States are separated into major divisions designated as "classes". There are five classes of air-cured tobacco, including light air-cured, dark air-cured, and three kinds of cigar tobaccos: filler, binder, and wrapper. Filler is the part which makes up the bulk of a cigar; binder is used to form the bunch and hold it in shape; while wrapper is used for the outside covering. Each of these tobaccos constitutes a type and is specially produced for the respective purpose. Under class, the subdivision is "types." Such classification is based on location of production, method of culture, and plant variety. Each tobacco type is further subdivided into grade groups which are named on the basis either of the principal use in manufacture or of stalk positions under the U.S. Government grading

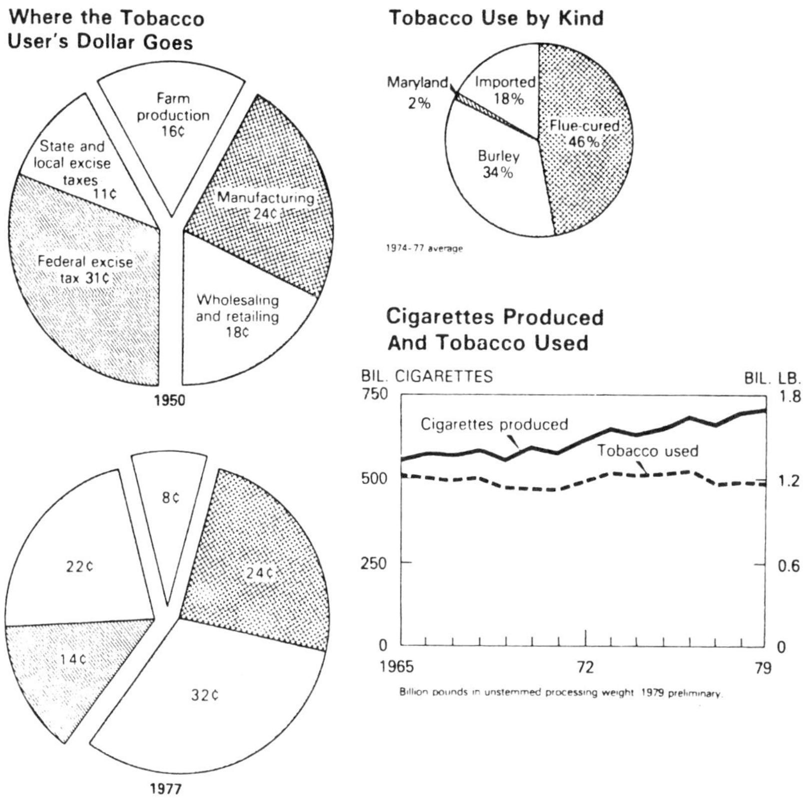

Figure 1. Left two economic "pies" show that the tobacco user's dollar goes mostly for manufacturing and wholesaling and retailing but taxes have decreased as has the farmer's return, 1950-77. Upper right "pie" shows the kind and source of tobacco being used. Lower right chart shows that cigarettes produced are increasing since 1965 in spite of total tobacco being used remaining about the same. This is due to use of stems, reconstituted sheets and filters in cigarette manufacture in recent years. (U.S.D.A.)

system. Each of the subdivisions is composed of a group of several grades, based on several elements of quality, such as body, texture, and color. However, tobacco farmers, leaf dealers, and manufacturers usually have their own grading system to meet their purposes.

In the United States, flue-cured is the most important domestic type, while Burley, a light air-cured type, is second in importance (Fig. 1).

Energy Requirement for Tobacco Production. To increase production efficiency, especially labor saving, much effort has been devoted to pest control, fertilizer, irrigation, growth regulation, and mechanization during field culture and the post harvest period. All this requires the use of energy, directly or indirectly. Cost of tobacco production varies from country to country because of the demand for energy, varying with locality. Those countries having hand laborers available and using less chemicals for tobacco production are, of course, comparatively lower in demand for fossil fuel energy. In the United States, flue-cured tobacco is the highest in energy demand per ace per year in comparison with any other crop, as shown in Table 1. The need of 20.8 barrels of oil equivalent to produce one acre of tobacco per year is almost 35 times the requirement of energy to produce one acre of wheat. This, of course, does not take into consideration the cash values of these two crops on a per acre basis.

Table 1. Comparative Energy Need for Production of Certain Crops in the United States.

Crop	Barrels of Oil/Acre/Year
Flue-cured tobacco	20.8
Tomato	18.9
Lettuce	15.0
Potato	9.6
Rice	8.2
Corn silage	4.1
Soybean	2.0
Wheat	0.6

Since 1964, when the U.S. Smoking and Health Report was released there has been continued increase in total units of cigarettes manufactured in the United States with some minor fluctuations from year to year. However, per capita consumption decreased from 11.53 lbs. in 1964 to 7.91 lbs. in 1979, and total tobacco consumption from 1.41 billion lbs. in 1964 to 1.1 billion lbs. in 1979. These facts can be explained by the recent usage in cigarette manufacture of stems, reconstituted sheets, and filters, and thus reduced the "waste" and increased the volume of the manufactured product (Figure 1).

American adults consumed less tobacco products per person in 1979 than they have since 1898, when chewing tobacco was more important than smoking tobacco. Chewing tobacco is showing a resurgence in recent years, according to Dr. Robert Miller, an economist with the U. S. Dept. of

Agriculture. Younger men have been attracted to chewing tobacco, apparently due to the media ads and TV portraying a rugged male chewing tobacco. A continuing drop in cigar and pipe smoking is predicted since urban and suburban lifestyle points more and more away from cigars and pipes, with smokers preferring a quick cigarette as the non-smoking areas proliferate.

Health Problems Associated With Tobacco Smoking

General Background. The association between tobacco smoking and health has been suggested and studied by many scientists during the past seventy years. The development of these smoking-health investigations may be arbitrarily divided into three periods. The first period, from 1900 to 1939, was primarily a period of statistical association. In 1900, an increase in lung cancer was noted in the vital statistics. Since then many studies were conducted on the possible relationships among tobacco smoking and cancer of the lung and of other organs, disease of the heart and blood vessels, and noncancer diseases of the lower respiratory tract. In 1939, F. H. Muller's report was published indicating a statistically significant correlation between cigarette smoking and lung cancer. The second period, from 1940 to 1963, was a period of more detailed cause-control investigations. In this period, many significant developments took place. In addition to further accumulation of statistical information, several large-scale cause-control studies were published, and many compounds in tobacco and tobacco smoke were isolated, identified, and some of them tested on experimental animals or tissues. It was established that application of cigarette smoke condensate tar resulted in extensive production of skin cancer in mice. The third or present period, beginning in 1964, is a period for the development of safer smoking products. In 1964, the report by the U. S. Surgeon General's Advisory Committee on Smoking and Health was published. It concluded that "cigarette smoking is casually related to lung cancer in men," and "cigarette smoking is a health hazard of sufficient importance in the United States to warrant appropriate remedial action." This report attracted public attention and led to the initiation of large-scale programs in tobacco health-related research. Several consecutive reports were published later by the U. S. Public Health Service confirming the earlier findings. More recent findings are summarized under various disease categories.

A 15-yr study reported in 1979 by the State Mutual Life Assurance Co. of America, Worcester, Mass., concluded that mortality rates for smokers (identical age and sex) were 2 to 4 times higher than for non-smokers. This was too great a difference to be ignored by life insurance underwriters.

The beneficial effects of smoking, however, should also be considered, especially in the area of mental health. These benefits originate in the psychogenic search for contentment and are measurable only in terms of

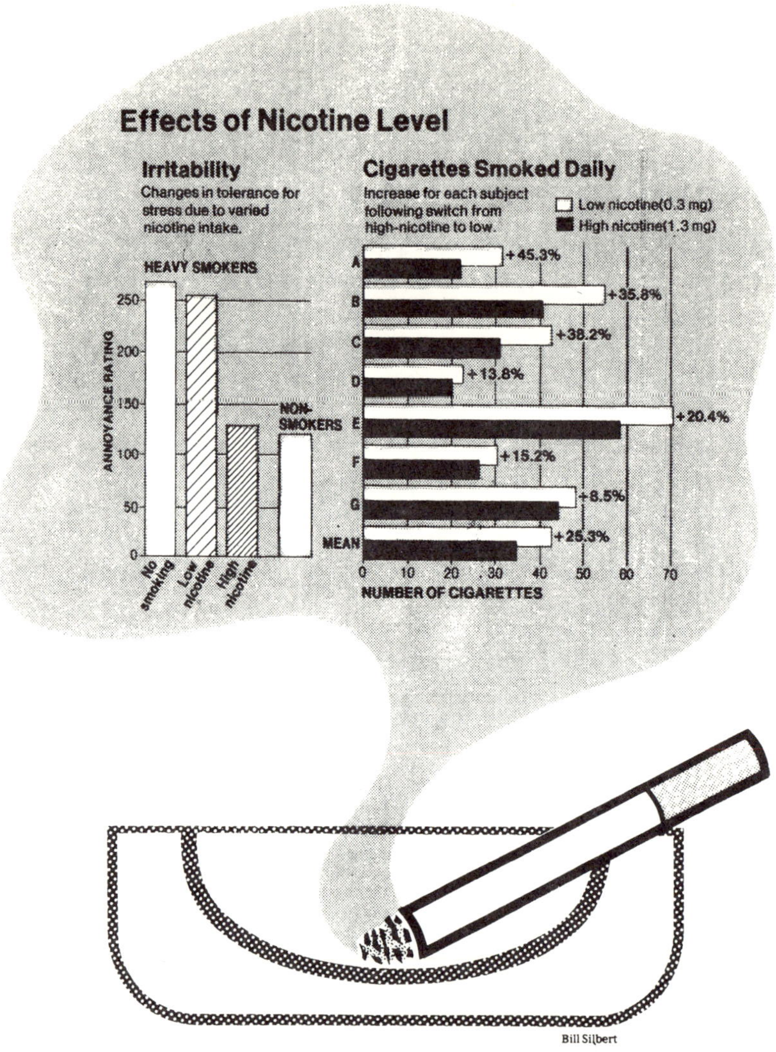

Figure 2. Dr. Stanley Schachter, professor of social psychology at Columbia University, New York City, found that heavy smokers have the least tolerance for "obnoxious noises" when not allowed to smoke. A low-nicotine cigarette helped a little, but the heavy smokers performed best on their own brand. He also found that people smoked more cigarettes per day when they were switched to a low-nicotine brand. Too, on a low-nicotine brand they seem to draw on them harder and hold the smoke in longer to maintain a desired level of nicotine in their blood. Thus, they may raise their intake of carbon monoxide, hydrogen cyanide and nitrogen oxides which are gasses implicated in cardiovascular disease, respiratory problems and fetal damage. (Bill Silbert and New York Times)

individual behavior. In a recent study on "the psychological dynamics of smoking" in the English population, it was concluded that "cigarettes are an important form of external effect control when there is inadequate internal control to cope with either high levels of stress or low threshold for affective arousal."

Relationship of Smoking and Cardiovascular Diseases.

a. Data from recent cause-effect studies suggest that cigarette smoking acts independently of and in conjunction with certain cardiac arrhythmias to increase the risk of mortality from coronary heart disease in men. Smokers also have a greater probability of dying from coronary heart disease (CHD) at an earlier age than nonsmokers. Women who smoke cigarettes have a greater risk of sudden death from CHD than do nonsmoking women.

b. Data from one recent incidence study suggest that cigarette smokers are more likely to develop hypertension than are nonsmokers. There is some evidence that suggests that stopping smoking may be accompanied by a rise in blood pressure.

c. The results of experimental studies demonstrate that the elevated levels of carboxyhemoglobin frequently seen in smokers may result in significantly decreased cardiac work performance and precipitation of ischemic electrocardiographic changes and arrhythmias in patients with clinical and subclinical CHD. Carboxyhemoglobin levels may be of value in determining a person's risk of developing arteriosclerotic cardiovascular disease.

d. Findings from experimental studies confirm that nicotine acts indirectly to cause elevations of the plasma free fatty acids (FFAs). The relative role of sympathetic versus adrenocortical stimulation of the rise in FFAs remains to be determined.

e. Cause-effect data reveal strong associations between cigarette smoking and development of peripheral vascular disease.

f. Data from cause-effect studies support a strong association between atherosclerotic brain infarction and cigarette smoking in premenopausal women and in men of all ages.

g. Carbon monoxide at levels of exposure commonly reached by cigarette smokers has been shown to decrease cardiac contractility in persons with coronary heart disease. Carbon monoxide has been shown to produce changes like those of early atherosclerosis in the aortas of rabbits.

Relationship of Smoking and Cancer.

a. Recent cause-effect evidence confirms the finding that cigarette smoking is the major cause of lung cancer for both men and women. Even in the presence of a possible genetic susceptibility to the development of lung cancer, cigarette smoking remains the major cause of lung cancer.

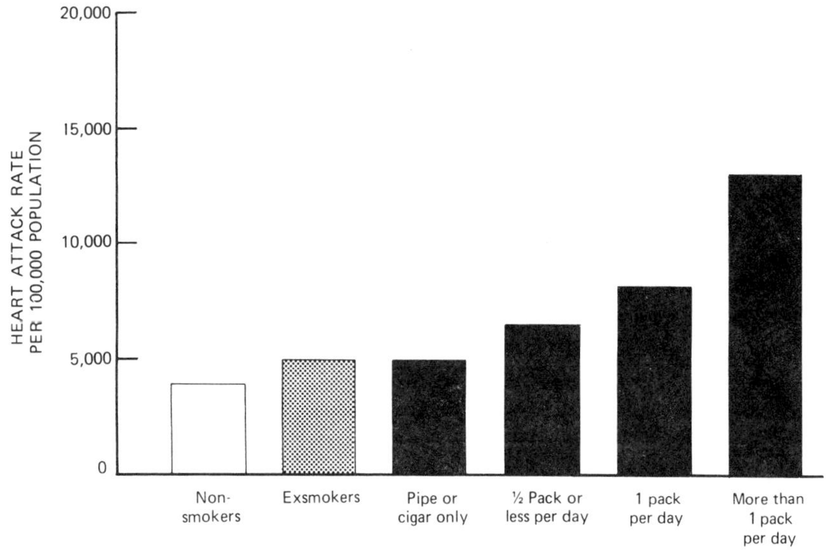

Figure 3. Chart shows the effect of smoking status on first heart attack of white males, 30-59 years of age, USA. (Nat. Cooperative Pooling Proj., Nat. Heart, Lung, Blood Inst., 1970.)

b. Filter cigarette smokers have a lower risk of developing lung cancer than nonfilter cigarette smokers, but that risk is still greater than the risk to nonsmokers and increases with increasing numbers of filtered cigarettes smoked.

c. Results from several studies demonstrated a dose-response relationship between smoking and oat cell carcinoma; a major prospective study demonstrated such a relationship for well-differentiated squamous cell carcinoma, oat cell carcinoma, and adenocarcinoma.

d. The current cause-effect data suggest that the incidence of lung cancer in women continues to rise. The rising incidence of lung cancer in women correlates well with the increasing trends in smoking among women.

e. Present data are conflicting with regard to dose-response relationships for cigar and pipe smokers and the development of lung cancer; the data are consistent for the fact that light cigar smokers are at a low risk of developing lung cancer.

f. Recent data confirm the synergistic effect of asbestos and smoking exposure on the risk of developing lung cancer in both men and women.

g. Results from experimental studies in hamsters continue to demonstrate that exposure to benzo(a)pyrene results in the production of respiratory tract malignancies, especially squamous cell carcinomas.

h. Data from experimental studies in animals suggest that chronic respiratory infections may enhance the carcinogenicity of components of cigarette smoke, as also may effect alterations in the immune system.

i. Current evidence suggests that components of cigarette smoke induce aryl hydrocarbon hydroxylase (AHH) activity in pulmonary macrophages in humans and in pulmonary parenchymal tissue and embryo cells in animals. Results from one study have shown that greater proportion of lung cancer patients had high levels of AHH activity than did healthy persons or persons with other cancers. Persons with high levels of AHH may be a group which has a genetically determined increased risk of lung cancer if they smoke, but no excess risk if they do not smoke.

j. Cigarette smoking and exposure to radioactivity by uranium miners have been related to cytologic changes in the respiratory tract epithelium including carcinoma in situ. Cigarette smoking has been more strongly related to these changes than exposure to mining-associated radioactivity.

k. Crysotile asbestos has been shown to contain traces of the carcinogen benzo(a)pyrene, and the combination of the two has been shown to be a more potent carcinogen in rats than either alone.

l. Recent epidemiologic data strongly indicate that cigarette smoking plays an independent role in the development of oral cancer. Heavy smoking before a first primary oral or respiratory cancer has been shown to be related to the development of a second primary in the respiratory tract or oral cavity.

m. Recent epidemiologic data confirm the association between smoking and pancreatic cancer.

n. Tobacco use seems to inhibit Vitamin C formation in the body.

Smoking and Non-Neoplastic Bronchopulmonary[2] Diseases.

a. Results from epidemiologic studies on elderly populations demonstrate an increased prevalence of respiratory symptoms and impairment of pulmonary lung function among smokers of both sexes compared with nonsmokers.

b. Data from several recent studies indicate that standard pulmonary function tests and physical work capacity are impaired in apparently healthy smokers compared with nonsmokers.

c. Recent epidemiologic data suggest that smokers who retain their cigarettes in their mouths continuously while smoking (''droopers'') have a higher prevalence of chronic bronchitis than those smokers who remove the cigarette from their mouths between puffs.

d. A recent epidemiologic study confirms the observation that cigarette smoke and air pollution act together to enhance the development of symptoms of respiratory disease.

---

[2]There is no abnormal growth or tumor in the lungs, as defined here.

e. Results from several recent studies indicate that cigarette smokers have a higher prevalence of functional abnormalities of the small airways than do nonsmokers.

f. Results from a recent study suggest that although a history of lower respiratory disease as an infant is related to the prevalence of cough at age 20, cigarette smoking is a far more important factor in the development of cough in young adulthood.

g. Data from a major retrospective study indicate that cigarette smoking is related to the development of bulbous (vesicles) disease of the lung.

h. Experimental studies in animals have shown that exposure to nitrogen dioxide, a constituent of the vapor phase of cigarette smoke, results in emphysema-like changes in the pulmonary parenchyma, diminished mucociliary clearance, and impairment of bactericidal activity of alveolar macrophages.

i. Data from experimental studies have demonstrated that the filtered gas phase of tobacco smoke may effect changes in pulmonary alveolar macrophage metabolism through inhibition of the pinocytotic pathway; cigarette smoke may also impair oxygen consumption and pinocytotic activity of pulmonary alveolar macrophages.

j. Pulmonary macrophages from cigarette smokers' lungs have a decreased ability to respond to *in vitro* antigenic stimuli as compared with macrophages from nonsmokers.

In 1979, 15 years after the original 1964 report, a new Surgeon General's Report on Smoking and Health was issued. Three major dangers were pointed out in this new report, including:

a. Mothers, who smoke during pregnancy face the possibility of creating long-term, irreversible effects on their babies. And as smoking levels among women go up, disease and death rates go up also: lung cancer has increased fivefold among women since 1955. Women who smoke like men die like men who smoke. Lung cancer in women is overtaking breast cancer.

b. Increased risks to smokers exposed to certain occupational hazards — workers in the asbestos, rubber, coat, textile, uranium, and chemical industries, among others, face these risks.

c. Smoking among children — the percentage of girls ages 12 to 14 who smoke, for example, has increased eightfold since 1968. Among the age group 13 to 19, there are now 6 million regular smokers. One hundred thousand children under 13 are regular smokers.

Toxic Components From Tobacco

Aflatoxin B_1, the most toxic of the four common aflatoxins, is produced by *Aspergillus flavus*. The binding of aflatoxin B_1 to both native and denatured DNA (deoxyribose nucleic acid) partially explains its extreme toxicity and carcinogenicity. Aflatoxins have been reported to occur in many commodities, but its presence in leaf tobacco has not been positively confirmed, although *A. flavus* was found in various grades of air-cured Burley tobacco. Certain types of tobacco contain higher populations of fungi than other types (Fargacs and Carll, 1966). These differences probably are the result of culture, and handling practices as well as chemical composition of tobacco leaf. Seven samples of good-grade cured tobacco from flue-cured, Burley, and Maryland types, and four samples of moldy tobaccos from flue-cured type, were used for aflatoxin studies. An examination of these samples of leaf tobacco and of cigarette smoke condensate, failed to detect aflatoxin B_1. Pure aflatoxin B_1 added to cigarettes was not recovered in the smoke condensate indicating that aflatoxin B_1, even if present, was changed or decomposed during the smoking process.

In a separate study conducted at the University of Kentucky, pregnant pigs were fed with tobacco stalks which had been exposed in the open field for several months. Baby pigs were found with abnormal development which possibly resulted from toxic materials generated by microorganisms on the tobacco stalk.

Many other leaf components, especially nicotine, are toxic in free form. In the plant, they generally occur chemically bound and are in a physiologically inactive form. This fact, of course, does not mean that such components are "safe" for humans or animals.

Concentrated 40% nicotine sulphate, which is diluted for spraying and insect control, when left on the human skin for awhile will enter the skin and cause typical nicotine poisoning. Strong nicotine kills insects by a paralyzing action.

Many insects attack tobacco plants despite the fact that tobacco alkaloids are toxic. The "adaptation" of insects to tobacco alkaloids is a fascinating phenomenon. Green peach aphid is able to subsist on tobacco because it feeds in the phloem of the plant and avoids the nicotine-containing xylem. Tobacco hornworm may excrete nicotine without degradation. There was no evidence of metabolism of nicotine to less toxic metabolites after topical, injected, or ingested doses. Although nicotine was detected in the blood of the hornworm, a toxic amount did not accumulate at the site of action. A comparative study has been conducted on the physiological responses of the nicotine-tolerant hornworm and the nicotine-susceptible silkworm to this alkaloid. It was concluded that the susceptibility may be, in part, the result of a less efficient ion-impermeable barrier of the silkworm's nervous system.

Adaptation of insects to nornicotine also has been studied. The hornworm tolerates nornicotine through a mechanism similar to that by which it tolerates nicotine, by excretion of the intact compound. Several other insects, including flies, grasshoppers, tobacco flea beetle, and southern armyworm were found to metabolize nornicotine.

Leaf tobacco was extracted by many scientists with various solvents for toxicity studies. Solvents used included aqueous Ba(OH)2, n-hexane, petroleum ether, and ethanol. Most of the studies suggested that the extract may play a role in tumor promoting activity. Others reported that ''mouse skin papillomas'' have been produced upon application of tobacco extracts without previous application of initiators.

The Characteristics of Tobacco Smoke

Pathophysiological Effects of Certain Smoke Components

Trace amounts of certain smoke components have been shown to exhibit pathophysiological effects on various tissues and organ systems. Some of these components are well known, including nicotine and related alkaloids, polynuclear aromatic hydrocarbons, N-nitrosamines, and toxic gases such as CO, NO_x, and HCN. Many excellent review articles have been published on toxic and tumorigenic effects of tobacco smoke. The toxic agents in tobacco smoke have been classified into four categories, including: (a) tumorigenic agents in the gas phase, (b) initiating agents in the particulate phase, (c) co-carcinogenic agents in the particulate phase, and (d) organ specific carcinogens in particulates. The components were summarized as follows:

a. Tumorigenic agents in the gas phase. *Carcinogens:* volatile and non-volatile N-nitrosamines, hydrazines, vinyl chloride, and possibly others. *Tumor promoters:* formaldehyde. *Cilia toxic agents:* HCN, formaldehyde, acetaldehyde, and acrolein.

b. Tumor initiating agents in the particulate phase. Benzo(a)pyrene; 5-methylchrysine; dibenzo(a,h)anthracene; benzo(b)fluoranthene; Benzo(j)fluoranthene; Dibenzo(a,h)pyrene; Dibenzo(i)pyrene; Dibenzo(a,j)a-cridine, and other related compounds.

c. Co-carcinogenic agents in the particulate phase. *Neutral fraction:* Pyrene; fluoranthene; benzo(ghi)perylene; naphthalenes; 1-methylindoles; 9-methylcarbazoles; 4,4'dichlorostilbene and others. *Acid fraction:* catechol and other phenols.

d. Organ-specific carcinogens in particulate phase (based on experimental data only). *Esophagus:* N-nitrosonornicotine and possibly N-nitrosoanabasine and other unknown unsymmetrical nitrosamines. *Lung:* Po-210, nickel compounds, cadmiums, other unknowns. *Pancreas:* nitrosamines, other unknowns; *Kidney and bladder:* B-naphthylamine, x-amino-fluorene; x-aminostilbene, o-toluidine, other aromatic amines, o-nitrotoluene, nitrosamines, etc.

The Potential for Producing Safer Tobacco

In dealing with an organic material as complex as tobacco, there are limitations for possible changes. The biological interaction and metabolic balance within a plant system, the combustion products and their biological activity, and the quality factors required for consumer acceptance are of equal importance. Our goal is to develop a tobacco which can satisfy farmers, manufacturers, and consumers in quality as well as in health aspects.

The task of developing a safer tobacco will be difficult and challenging, but the potential is great. Preliminary findings are encouraging. There are opportunities for genetic changes and improvements in cultural and curing practices. For example, current knowledge on the inheritance of alkaloids in the tobacco plant is well advanced. It is possible to breed tobacco varieties with a wide range of nicotine content. Next to nicotine, among the most commonly found alkaloids in tobacco are nornicotine, anatabine, and anabasine. New strains of tobacco plants with extremely low or high levels of nicotine are available. Similarly, various levels of phytosterols, polyphenols, lipids, other nitrogenous compounds and carbohydrates can be produced in leaf tobacco through genetic, agronomic, cultural and biochemical regulation.

A new curing process, homogenized leaf curing (HLC) has been developed. This procedure involves homogenization, incubation and dehydration. At the "slurry" state, desired chemical composition can be achieved by controlled enzyme action; undesirable components can be removed by extraction. Physical properties can be improved by sheet reconstitution of desired porosity and thickness. *Preliminary results demonstrated that cigarettes processed by HLC may provide smoke with quality comparable to that from conventionally cured leaf, but with much lower biological response.*

Modification of Tobacco Products. In attempting the development of a less hazardous cigarette, many experimental products were made and detailed chemical and biological tests were consulted. Some of the results are as follows. Smoke condensate from experimental cigarettes made with high porosity paper, or with tobacco stems (midribs), or with reconstituted sheets were less tumorigenic than condensates from regular tobacco. Condensate from cigarettes made of tobacco laminae was very toxic. Neither the width of tobacco cuts nor the addition of nitrates appeared to affect the condensate tumorigenicity.

The low nicotine/normal fertilizer and low nicotine/high fertilizer blends showed significantly lower tumorigenicity than normal nicotine/normal fertilizer blends. There were no significant differences, however, between the low nicotine/normal fertilizer and low nicotine/high fertilizer blends. Several methods of treating cured leaf tobacco, including puffing, expansion and freeze-drying did not show significant differences among themselves. However, expansion and freeze drying showed significantly lower condensate tumorigenicty than did the controls. For artificial tobacco substitutes, one had the lowest condensate tumorigenicity and the other had the highest among the blends tested.

For sucker agent fatty alcohol treatment, the normal residue level (4.8 ppm), and 100 times enriched level (480 ppm) and hand-suckered blends showed no differences compared to controls. Additives, casing materials, dilution filters all showed considerable effects in smoke constituents.

The results of the correlation analysis of several constituents of leaf tobacco, smoke constituents, and biological activity were studied. The concentrations of both nicotine and tar, as constituents of the condensate, were highly correlated with the incidence of tumorigenicity on mouse skin. Static burn rate was negatively correlated with tumorigenic activity. Other compounds that were negatively correlated with tumorigenicity were acetaldehyde, formaldehyde, NO_x, CO, and acrolein. Total phenolics in the leaf, H_2O per cigarette and benz(a)anthracene in the condensate were positively correlated with tumorigenicity.

Beneficial Byproducts From Tobacco

Food Source. Among all the components in tobacco only a small portion is essential for smoke quality and desirability. Others are either inert materials which do not have any effect on tobacco usage or are components which serve as precursors of undesirable smoke constituents. The latter two groups of components are literally "wasted" during combustion and could be used for feed or food.

If the usable proteins are removed for food in tobacco it would be sufficient to feed 34 to 63 million people, depending on the diet standard required.

Pesticides, medicinal and industrial use. For many years, nicotine from tobacco was one of the most important insecticides. "Black Leaf 40" contained 40% (by weight) of nicotine in the form of nicotine sulfate. In earlier days, Black Leaf 40 was even used for "Official dipping" treatment of animals for scabies, lice, sheep ticks, etc. Nicotine has not been widely used for such practices since the production of the synthetic organic phosphate pesticides. This change, however, does not reduce the economic value of nicotine itself. Nicotine, in fact, will be in higher demand should the total synthetic "tobacco" become a reality.

Tobacco stalks can be used for fertilizer, fuel, compost, livestock bedding, paper manufacture, fiberboard, or insulating board. Oil has been extracted from tobacco seed. Soap has been made from tobacco fat, and waxes may be produced from tobacco extracts. Tobacco "essence" was collected for its characteristic aroma. Tobacco is known as a possible source of many chemicals, including nicotine, nicotinic acid, rutin, pectin, and certain organic acids. Rutin, of course, is well known for its medical use in strengthening capillary blood vessels.

Recent developments in sheet reconstitution in the tobacco industry make use of all tobacco matrials which years ago were considered as "waste". Such materials not only include "stems,""dust," or "siftings," but also tobacco stalks.

Considering the fact that tobacco is one of the highest energy demanding agricultural products, it is only reasonable that all tobacco materials should be used, especially those which are wasted through combustion.

THE NIGHTSHADES RESEARCH FOUNDATION

If you would like to contribute to the research efforts in the long neglected *human nutrition,* we would appreciate very much hearing from you. Most of the funds by far will go for research with relatively little for administration. Please contact the Foundation in care of the author of this book. Data already assembled from survey studies indicate that well over fifty percent of ill-health expenses today can be attributed directly or indirectly to the consumption and use of the nightshades.

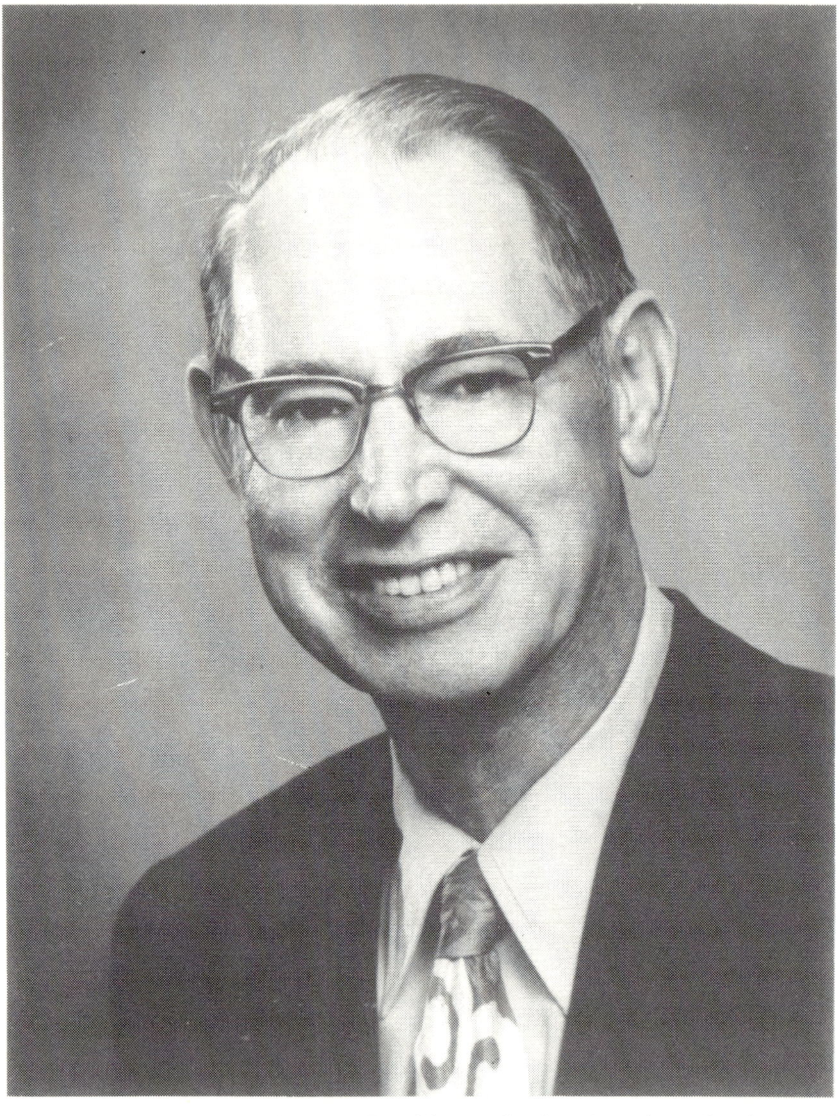

Dr. George Kelso Davis was President of The American Institute of Nutrition in 1975-6, dealing with both livestock and humans. In 1976-7 he held the office of President of The Society for Environmental Geochemistry and Health. His research interests since graduating from Cornell and Pennsylvania State Universities have been in nutrition and the development of diseases; trace mineral substances, radioactive tracers and copper and cardiovascular disorders, mainly in livestock. His accompanying Chapter explains the effects of livestock feeding on the nightshade, *Solanum malacoxylon,* which is the same genus as the white potato, *Solanum tuberosum* and the eggplant, *Solanum Melongena.*

CHAPTER VI

Effect of a Nightshade on Livestock

By George K. Davis
Professor of Nutrition
University of Florida, Gainesville, Fla. 32601

For at least ninety-five years, there has existed in the breeding zone of the Province of Buenos Aires a condition of cattle that has resulted in losses of about 10% of the population each year. This has been caused by a disease which is endemic in the zone and generally called "enteque seco". The economic loss which is due to morbidity is certainly much greater than that which is due to mortality. The characteristics of the disease are lack of appetite, loss of weight, increase of calcium and phosphorus in the blood and lesions of the soft tissues, primarily elastic fibers which are calcified, especially the calcification of the cardiovascular system. In 1967, B. J. Carrillo and N. A. Worker determined that by forced consumption of the leaves of a nightshades *Solanum malacoxylon,* a calcification (hardening) of certain of the tissues of cattle could be caused. A water extract of the leaves of this plant contained the toxic principle, since feeding of this product caused the same lesions to develop in cattle as occurred when the leaves of the *Solanum malacoxylon* were fed.

The same or nearly identical pathology has been described by Dobereiner[1] and associates in Brazil where the common name is "Espichamento". In Hawaii the disease is called "Naalehu disease" and has been described by F. Lynd and co-workers. In Jamaica the condition has been called "Manchester wasting disease". In the European Alps "enzootic calcinosis" would appear to be a disease with similar pathology.

An attempt was made to produce the same characteristics in rats by using either the leaves or the water extract but without success. Later studies using an extract of *Solanum malacoxylon* and of an extract incubated with rumen fluid caused similar changes to occur in rats. The quantities used may have been a factor.

In the early experiments in Argentina, it was found possible to use either cattle or sheep and observe the increased level of calcium and/or phosphate in the blood serum as a measure of the toxicity of the *Solanum malacoxylon* which was being given to the animals. This rapidly was developed into an assay technique for evaluating the toxic principle.

---

[1]See first edition of this book for technical references supporting data and statements.

Blood Calcium

It was discovered that in cattle as little as 100 grams of dry *Solanum malacoxylon* leaves placed in the rumen through a fistula would result in an increase in blood calcium and phosphate approximating 50% of normal values within a period of 48 hours. Without subsequent administration of the plant material, the blood calcium and phosphate would return to normal in a period of approximately 72 hours.

It was possible to use a simple water extract of the leaves and cause the same elevation of blood calcium and phosphorus in either cattle or in sheep. In this way it was determined that the most toxic portion of the plant appeared to be the leaves.

It was a common observation that feeding the leaves of *Solanum malacoxylon* resulted in a rapid loss of appetite and only by force feeding could the animals be made to consume any appreciable quantity of the *Solanum* plant in feeding trials.

The failure to observe animals consuming leaves from plants when on pasture raised considerable doubt as to the relationship between the *Solanum malacoxylon* and the endemic soft tissue calcification observed in cattle and to some extent in sheep and horses in the areas where *Solanum malacoxylon* was observed to be abundant.

The problem of how the Solanum might cause the soft tissue calcification when the plant was obviously so unpalatable to the animals was finally solved when it was observed that the roots of the plant extend out from the base for up to 15 meters and that every node is a source of a small shoot coming up in the grass. Under these circumstances cattle and sheep and horses find it difficult or impossible to avoid consuming the plant when grazing.

Solanum malacoxylon occurs in low areas from Campo Grande, Brazil south to Bahia Blanca, Argentina. While most prevalent in low areas subject to flooding during periods of heavy rainfall, it is not restricted to these areas but is found over much of the pasture land in that part of South America.

Solanum malacoxylon is a shrub that grows to between 1 and 1.5 meters in height. The stems are tall and smooth with leaves that are sharp pointed on fairly long stems and characterized as somewhat fleshy and peach like. The plant is generally a light green color.

The occurrence of the soft tissue calcification has been reported in all of the areas where the plant is known to grow but is much more severe during periods of drought. While the plant grows in much of the so called breeding area of Buenos Aires province, it is more abundant in the low lying areas and consequently with dry weather and the animals forced to seek forage in the lower areas, the exposure to the plant is much greater; and therefore, the occurrence of the condition known as "enteque seco" is much more frequent.

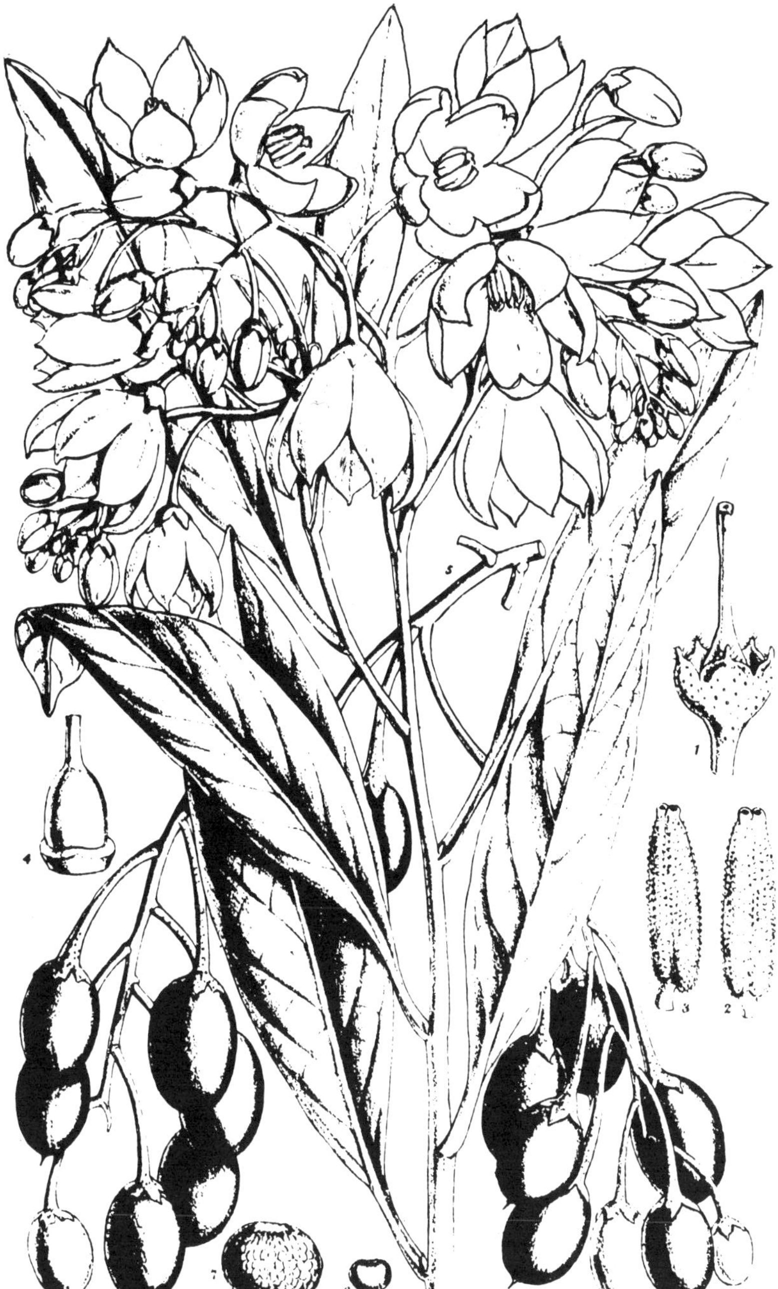

This is *Solanum malacoxylon,* a nightshade, on which the cattle in Argentina fed in the pastures, causing the so-called ''Entique seco'' disease (locally), but in scientific literature is known as enzootic calcinosis. This nightshade is of the same genus as the white potato, *Solanum tuberosum* and the eggplant, *Solanum Melangena.* (Courtesy of Royal Botanic Gardens, Kew, London, England).

Vitamin D Relationship

The similarity between the soft tissue calcification seen in cattle and sheep exposed to *Solanum malacoxylon* and soft tissue calcification caused by extremely high levels of *vitamin D* administered to animals experimentally suggested the possibility of a relationship. However, the very small amount of *Solanum malacoxylon* and the very rapid response in terms of elevated blood calcium and phosphate with calcification of the tissues, as compared with the rather lengthy time required for extremely high levels of vitamin D administered orally to cause the same kind of pathology, suggested that these two conditions were not the same.

Subsequent experiments with guinea pigs and with rabbits demonstrated that the water extract of *Solanum malacoxylon* caused a decrease in body weight gains, a reduction in feed and water consumption, and led to mortality. The post-mortem examination of guinea pigs treated with a water extract of the *Solanum* showed calcification of the aorta and cardiac muscle and of the intercoastal muscles. It was also noticed that contrary to the observation on cattle, there was calcification of the kidney tissues. The hypercalcemia and occasional hyperphosphatemia which occur suggested that the condition in guinea pigs was a parallel to that which was seen in animals in Argentina.

Still another observation was the fact that the magnesium level also was increased in these tissues indicating that magnesium absorption also had been increased by the water extract of the *Solanum malacoxylon.*

Although original work in Argentina did not show calcification of kidney tissues, subsequent work with sheep suggested that some animals there is a deposition of calcium phosphate in the kidney tubules. J. L. Evans and associates, Rutgers University, have found kidney stones in rats fed potatoes.

The occurrence of soft tissue calcification and particularly the deposition of calcium phosphate in the cardiovascular tissues has led to a close examination of the progress of this condition. The early observations that a copper deficiency resulted in a degradation of the elastic fibers of the cardiovascular system led to an examination of the copper status of cattle in the area where the soft tissue calcification was occurring. This led to the discovery that cattle suffering from the "enteque seco" frequently showed very low copper values in the liver and were apparently suffering from a copper deficiency. This copper deficiency did not appear to be paralleled by a molybdenum toxicity as has been reported in Florida and other parts of the world.

It appeared that the copper deficiency might cause a breakdown of elastic fibers providing a focus for the deposition of the calcium phosphate and perhaps explaining the selectivity of the disease for the cardiovascular system.

It should be observed that while the elastic fibers of the cardiovascular system were affected early in the disease other tissues including those of the lung, diaphragm, and ligamentum nuchae (neck) were also noted to be heavily calcified in long standing cases of "enteque seco" in cattle.

The demonstration by workers at Wisconsin, Arizona and Cornell that the metabolism of orally ingested vitamin D_3 followed a pathway from intestinal absorption to the liver where 25 hydroxycholecaciferol is formed, to the kidney where 1a[1], 25 dehydroxycholecalciferol, the active form of vitamin D_3 is formed. The active form functions as a hormone stimulating the formation of calcium binding protein. The protein transports calcium across the gut membranes and phosphate absorption also appears to be increased.

Normally, orally ingested vitamin D and that found in the body by ultraviolet irradiation is subject to homeostatic control through the action of parathormone and calcitonin but when the active form 1a $25(OH)_2D_3$ is consumed as part of the diet, these controls are bypassed and as a result abnormal amounts of the transport protein, CaBP, are formed and calcium absorption is stimulated.

Dr. Robert Wasserman and his colleagues at Cornell University have demonstrated that the active principle of vitamin D is present not only in *Solanum malacoxylon*[2] but also in *Cestrum diurnum*[2] a plant growing in many tropical and subtropical areas and in *Tricetum flavescens*[3], a grass, growing in the German Alps perhaps in a slightly different form.

This demonstration that the active form of vitamin D is present in at least three species of three different genera of plants, raises many questions regarding the possible role of diet and calcium and phosphorus metabolism. Are there many other plants common to human diets as well as animal feeds that contain significant if small quantities of the active form of vitamin D? Can the presence of such a compound be used advantageously to protect against the occurrence of osteomalacia? Is is possible that the presence of the active form of vitamin D may result in abnormal calcium absorption and deposits in connective tissue with resultant pathology?

Obviously the discovery that plants can form the active vitamin D_3 opens a vast new area of research with potentially far reaching importance for human and animal health.

---

[1]a refers to alpha, [2]Nightshades, [3]Gramineae

Are You Really On The No-Nightshades Diet?

The Following Photographs

The following photographs show the effects of livestock feeding on nightshade plants. The bone, tendon and tissue breakdown are similar to that found in certain forms of arthritis and other disease problems in humans. References to these research efforts can be found in the first edition of this book.

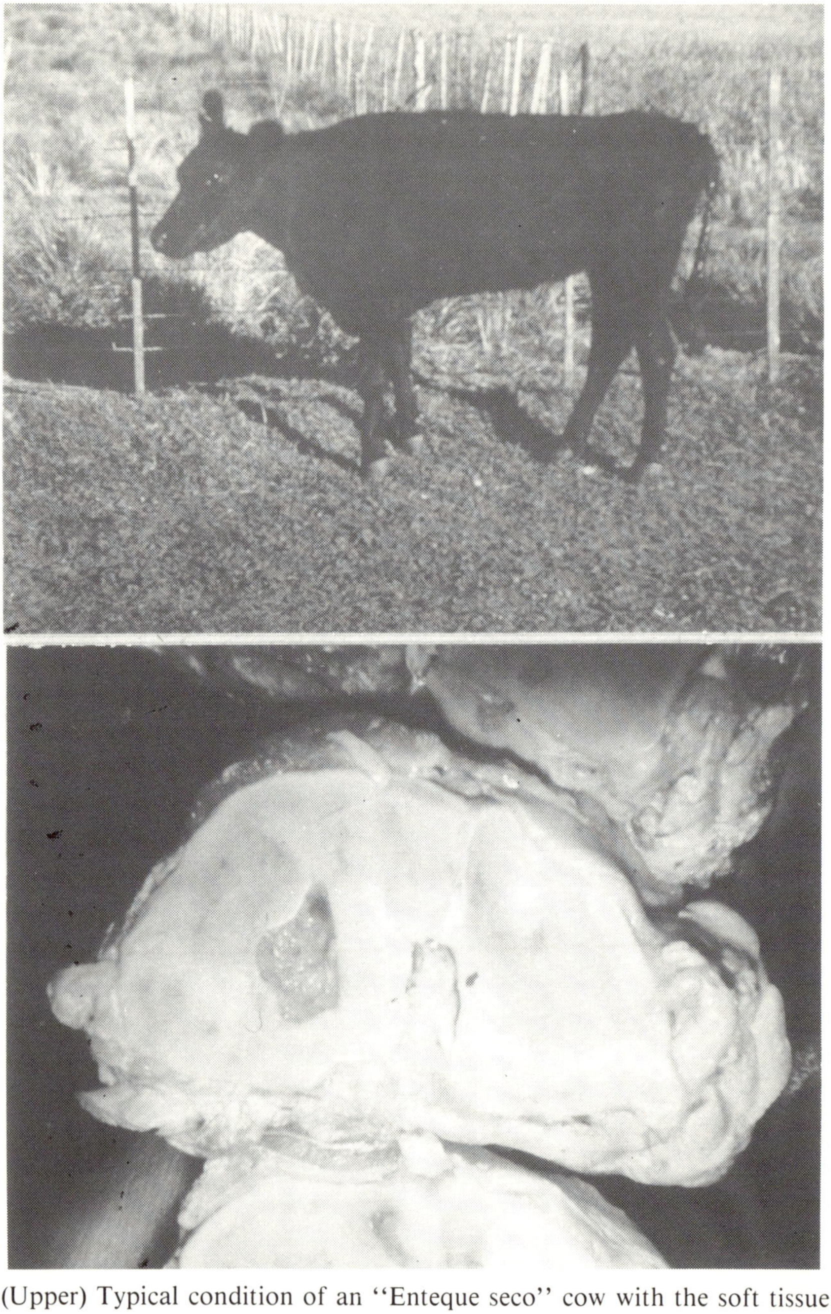

(Upper) Typical condition of an "Enteque seco" cow with the soft tissue (cardiovascular and lung) calcification causing the wasting symptoms and pathology. (Lower) Although the animals with this disease moved with obvious pain, the joints at this point showed only limited involvement. (G.K. Davis, Univ. of Fla.)

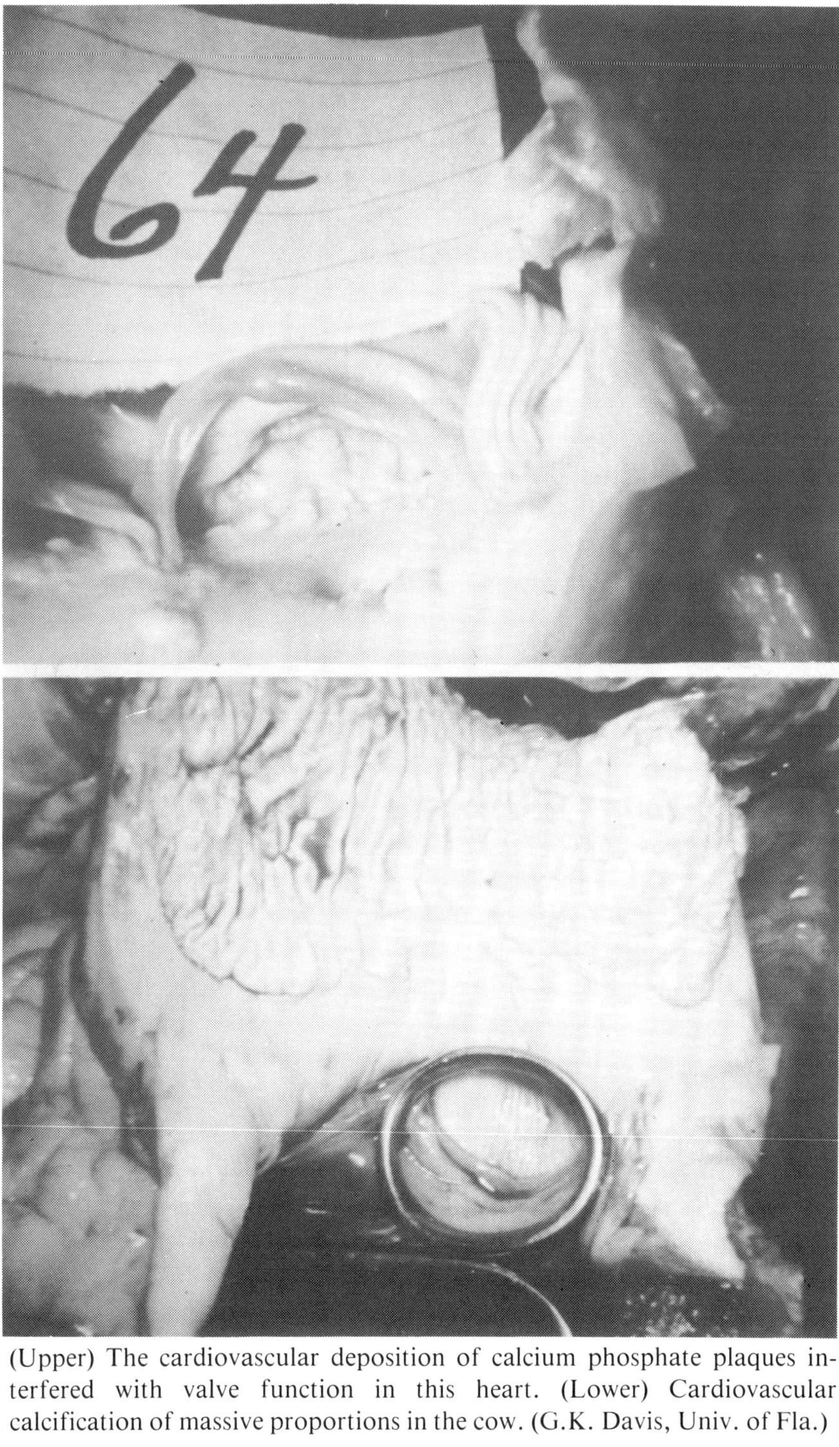

(Upper) The cardiovascular deposition of calcium phosphate plaques interfered with valve function in this heart. (Lower) Cardiovascular calcification of massive proportions in the cow. (G.K. Davis, Univ. of Fla.)

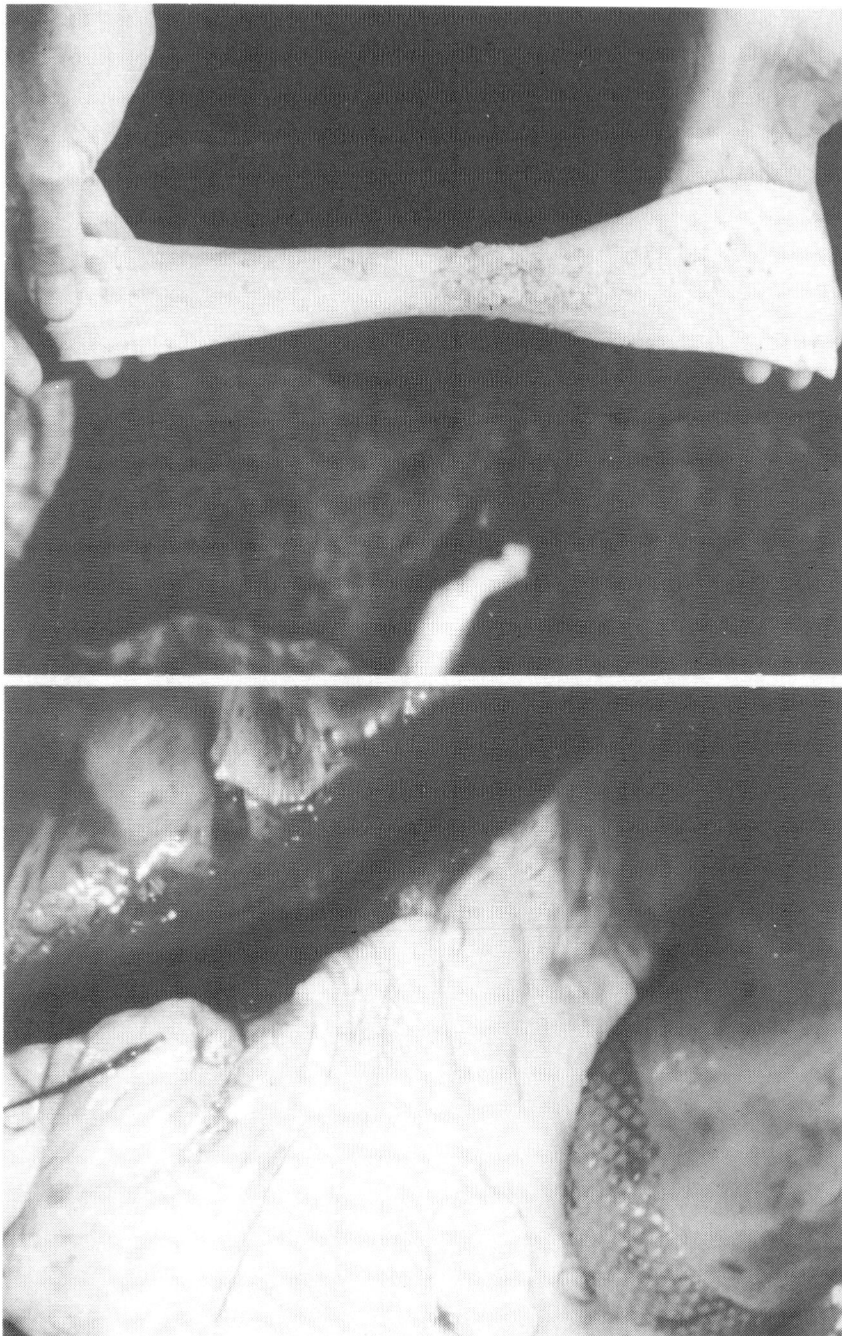

(Left) This shows calcification of the coronary arteries. (Right) Calcification of the large aorta of the "Entique" cow. (G.K. Davis, Univ. of Fla.)

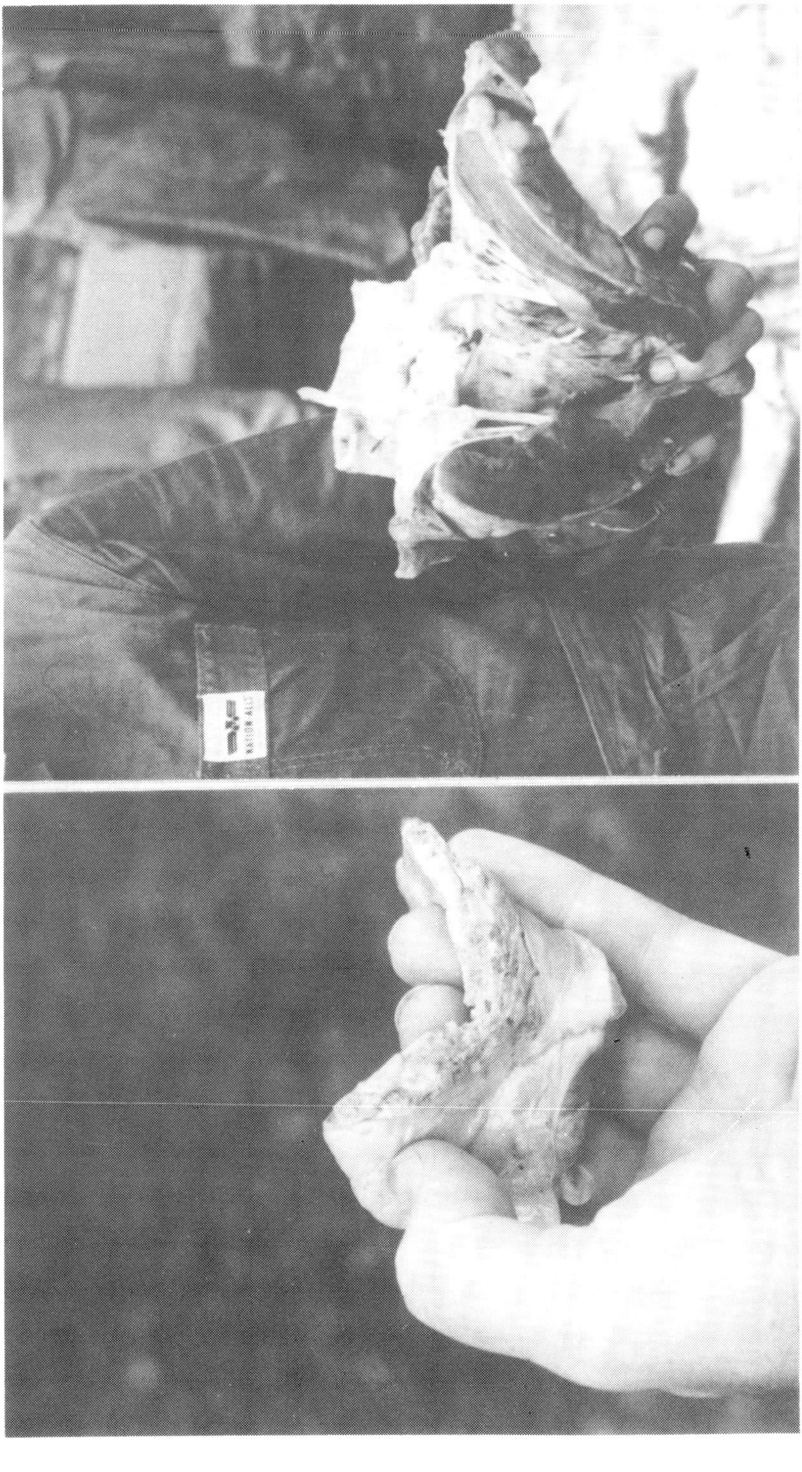

(Left) A calcified section of the lung of the cow. (Right) The calcified heart and aorta. (G.K. Davis, Univ. of Fla.)

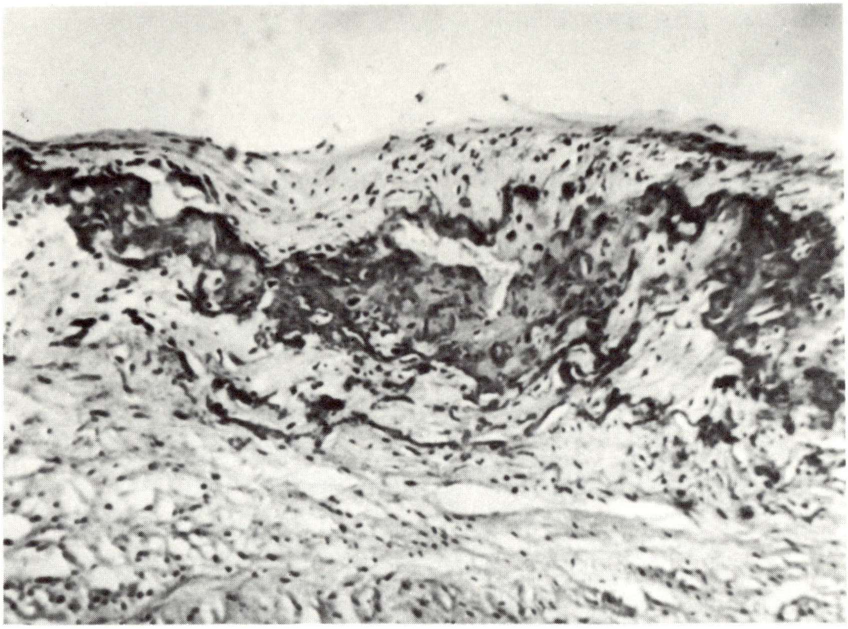

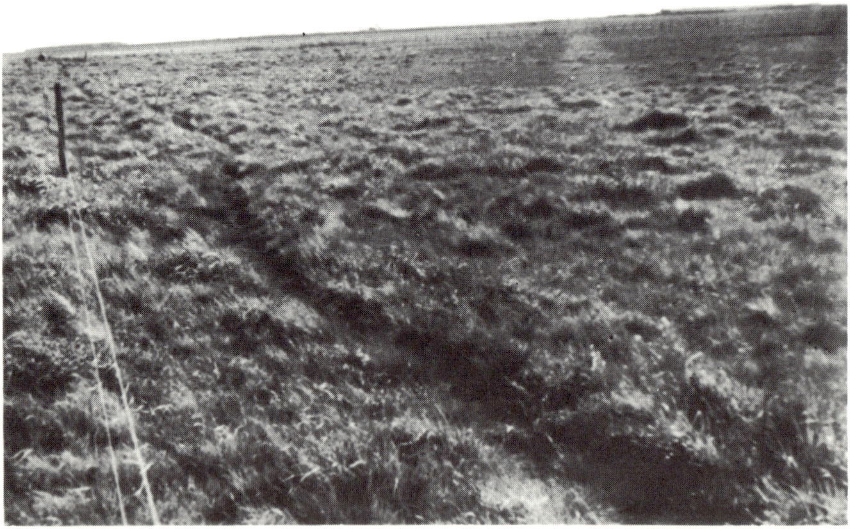

(Upper) An artery from the "Entique" cow with calcium plaque. (Lower) A typical pasture containing with the grass the *S. malacoxylon* nightshade weed that caused the "Entique seco" condition of the cattle. The cattle were found eating the tender shoots arising from extended underground roots of the nightshade plant. (G.K. Davis, Univ. of Fla.)

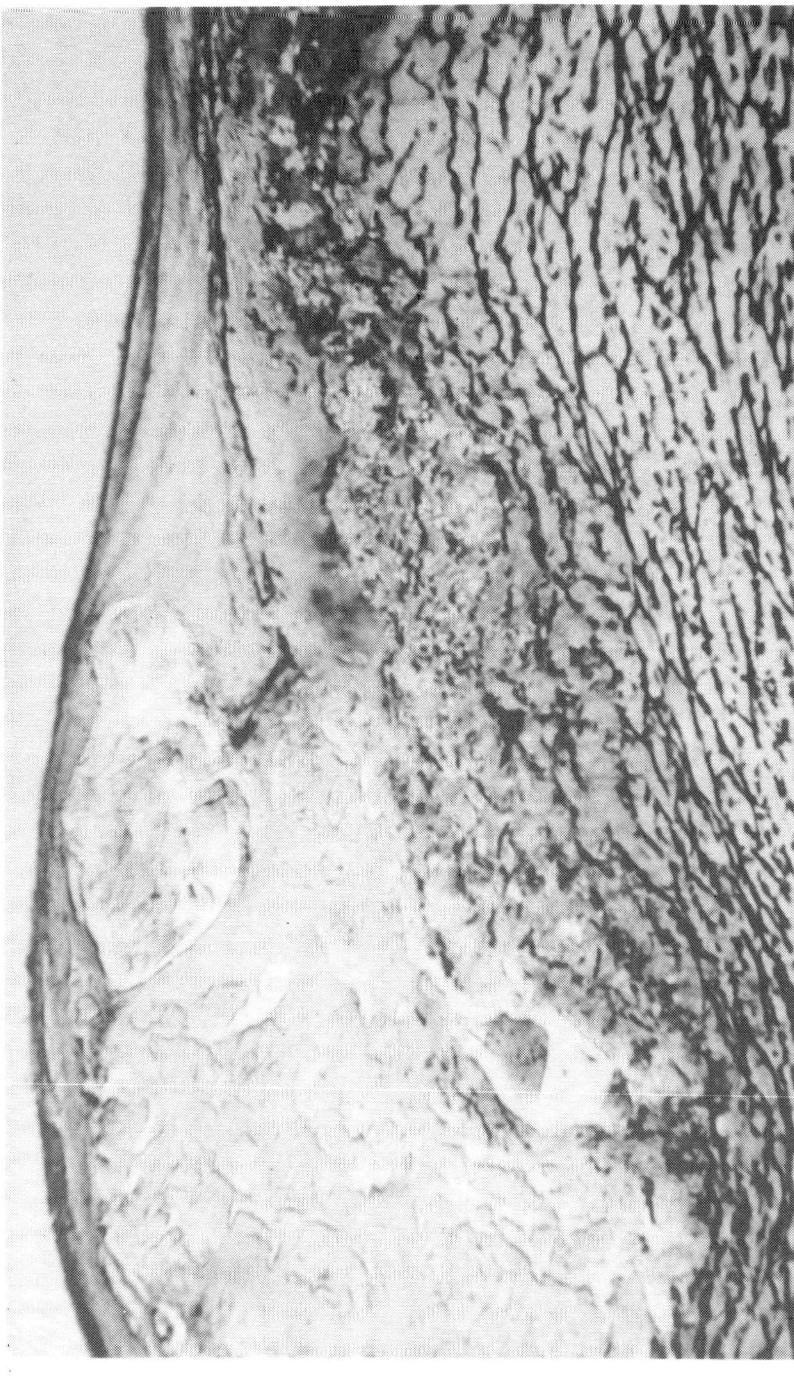

A microscopic section of the aorta near the heart of the cow showing the calcium phosphate deposit protruding into the lumen of the blood vessel. (G.K. Davis, Univ. of Fla.)

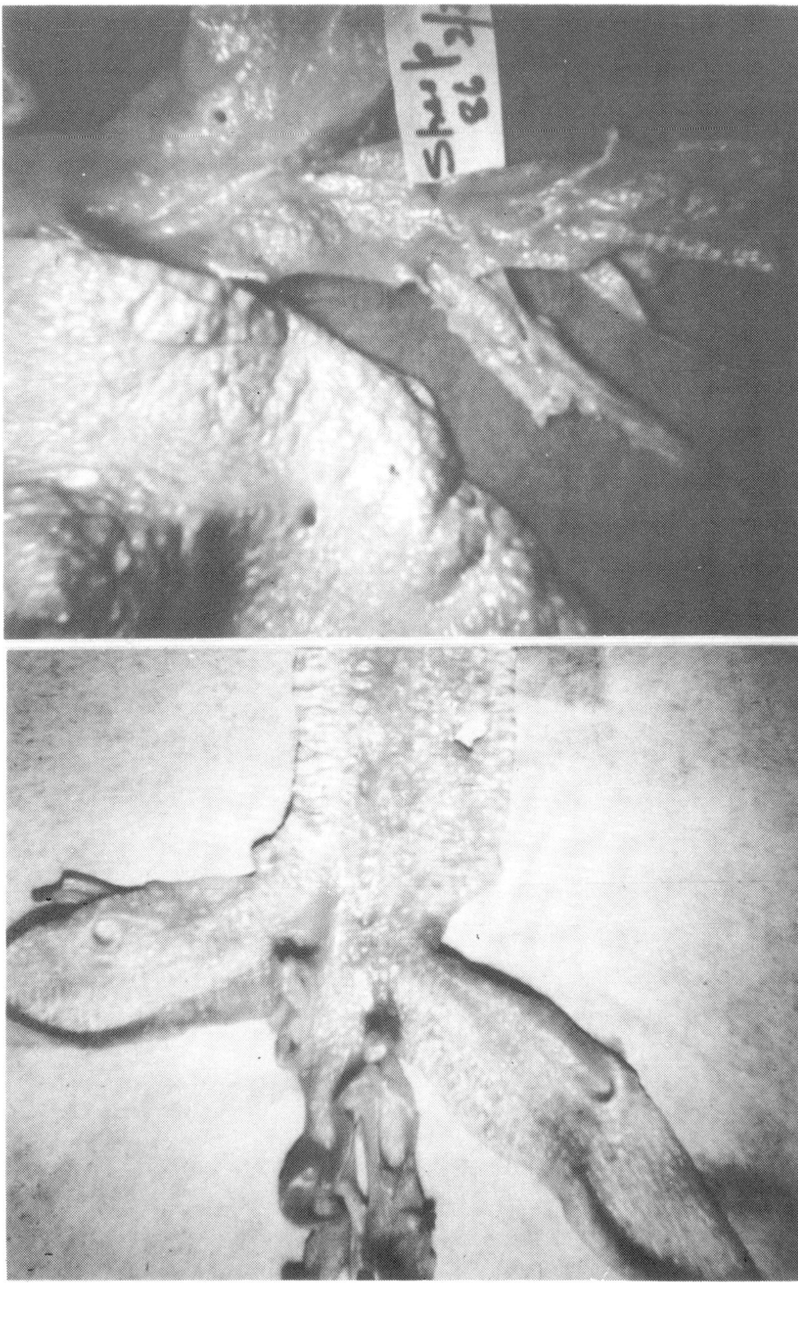

(Left) When extracts of *Solanum malacoxylon* are fed to sheep, there is rapid calcification of arteries. (Right) Massive calcification of the aorta develops as shown here.

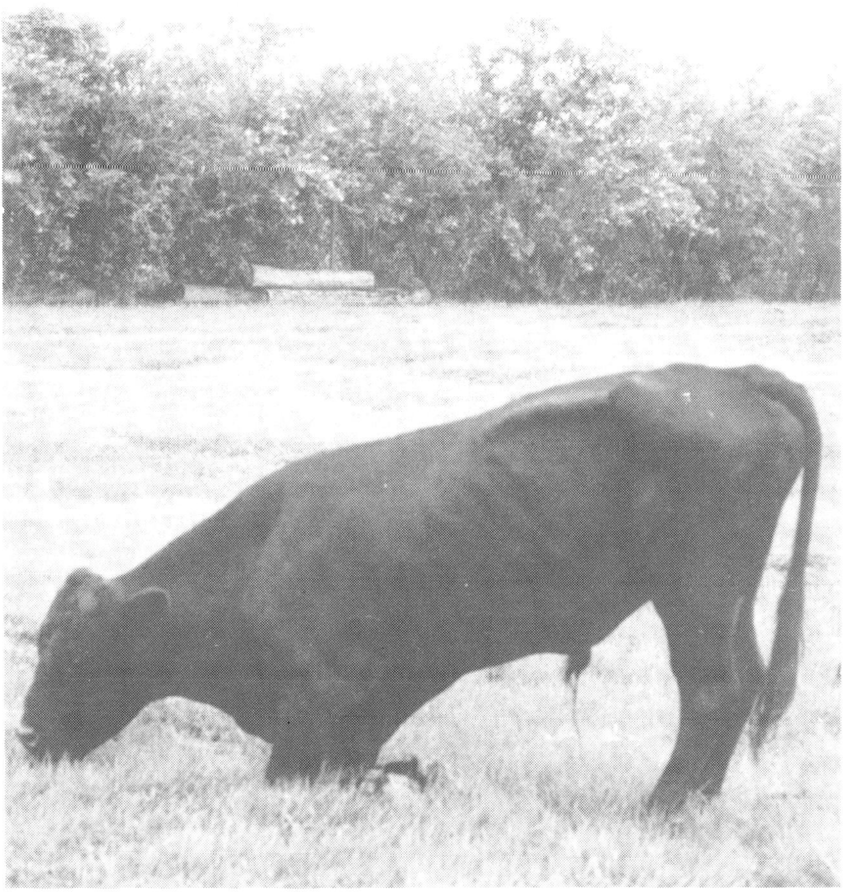

A three-year Aberdeen Angus bull in poor nutritional condition with visible ribs but alert with good appetite. Bull is grazing on its knees due to extremely tender flexor tendons and suspensory ligaments. A solid stand of the nightshade, *Cestrum diurnum,* Linn., can be seen along the background fencerow on which the bull also had been feeding, in Florida. It is reported that hogs fed an abundance of white potatoes in Germany may be seen feeding on their knees. (Photo courtesy Lennart Krook, Cornell University College of Veterinary Medicine, Ithaca, N.Y.)

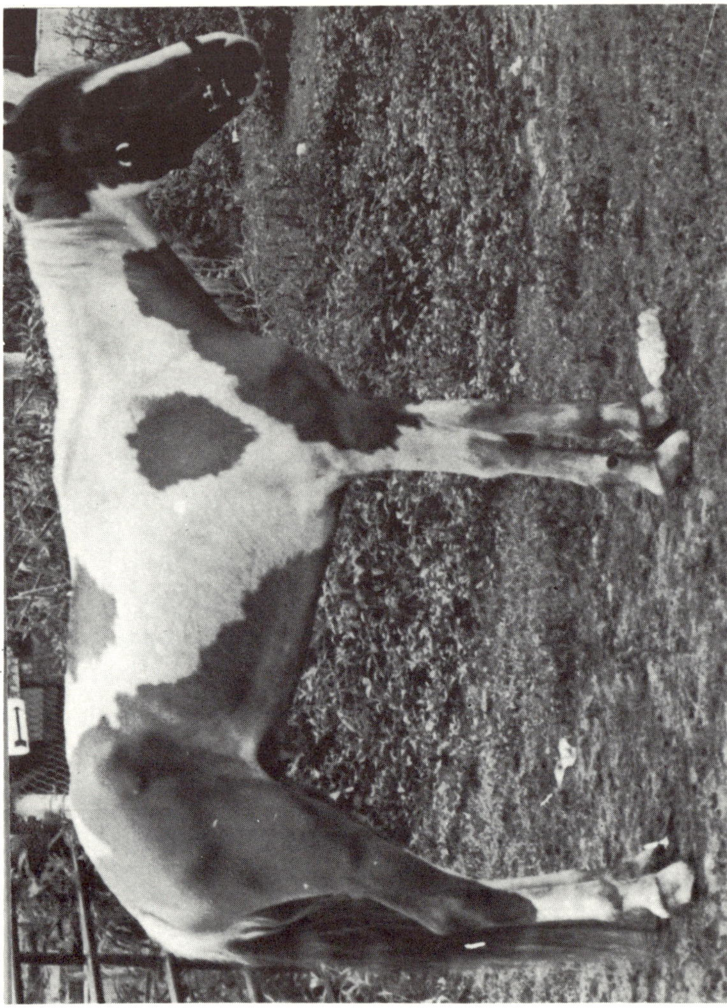

This three-year pony male shows chronic malformed legs and joints, general wasting, retracted abdomen and a slightly humped back, due to feeding on a fencerow nightshade, *Cestrum diurnum*, Linn., in Florida. (Courtesy R.H. Wasserman, Cornell University Veterinary College.)

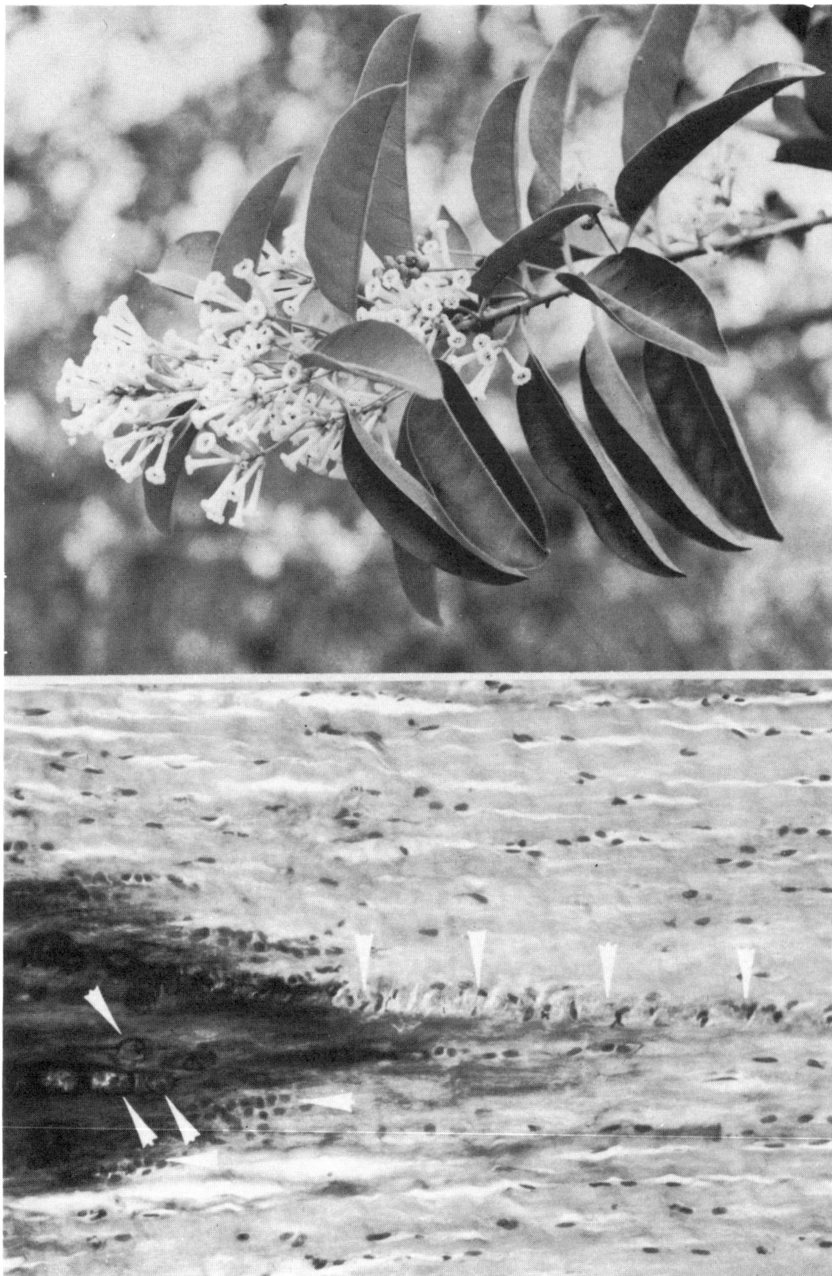

(Upper) The nightshade, *Cestrum diurnum,* known as Chinese inkberry, day-blooming jessamine, king-of-the-day, on which the pony and bull were feeding. (Lower) Degeneration of elastic fiber of suspensory ligament (center right) and mineralization at left of pony. (R. H. Wasserman, Cornell Veterinary College.)

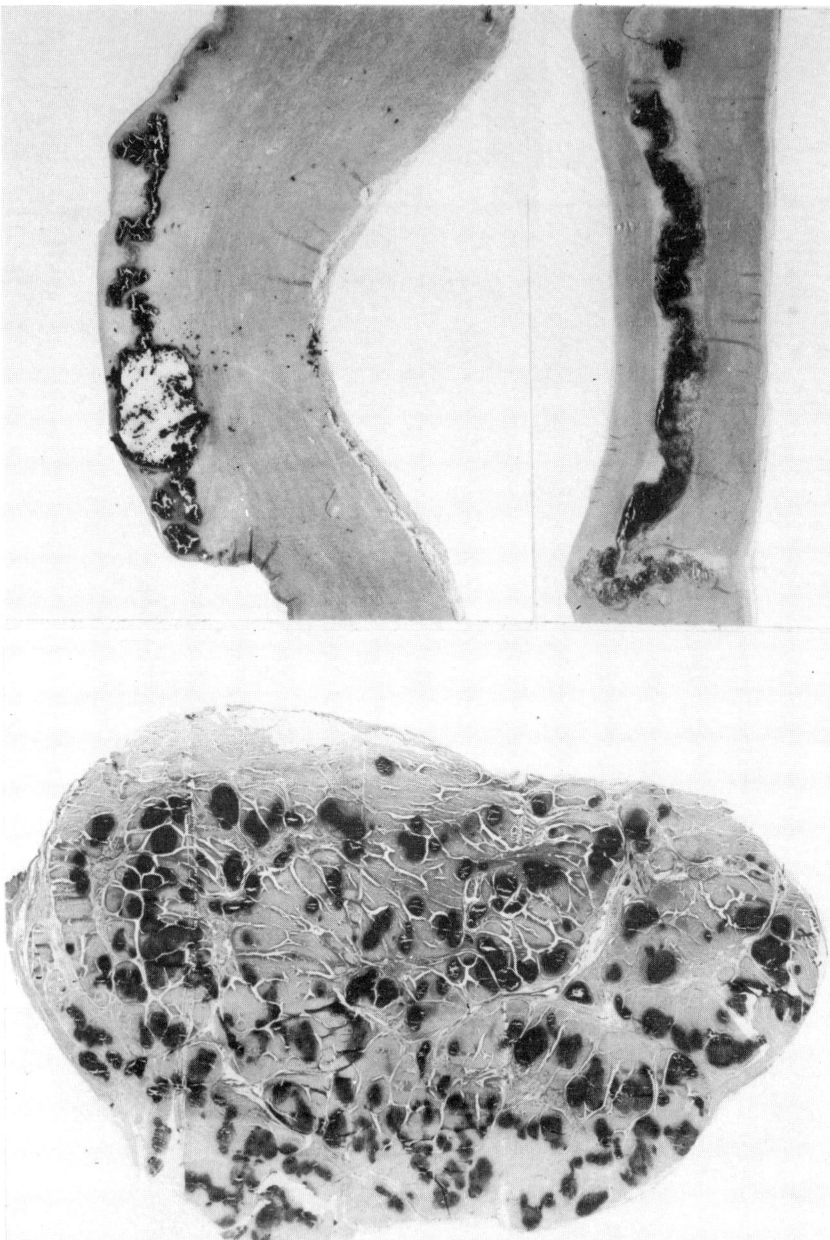

(Upper) At left is pony's aortic blood vessel wall just above aortic heart valves. At right is aortic arch wall, both walls showing extensive mineralized hardening after feeding on *C. diurnum*. (Lower) Mineralized dark areas in suspensory ligament of thoracic limb. (R.H. Wasserman, Cornell Veterinary College).

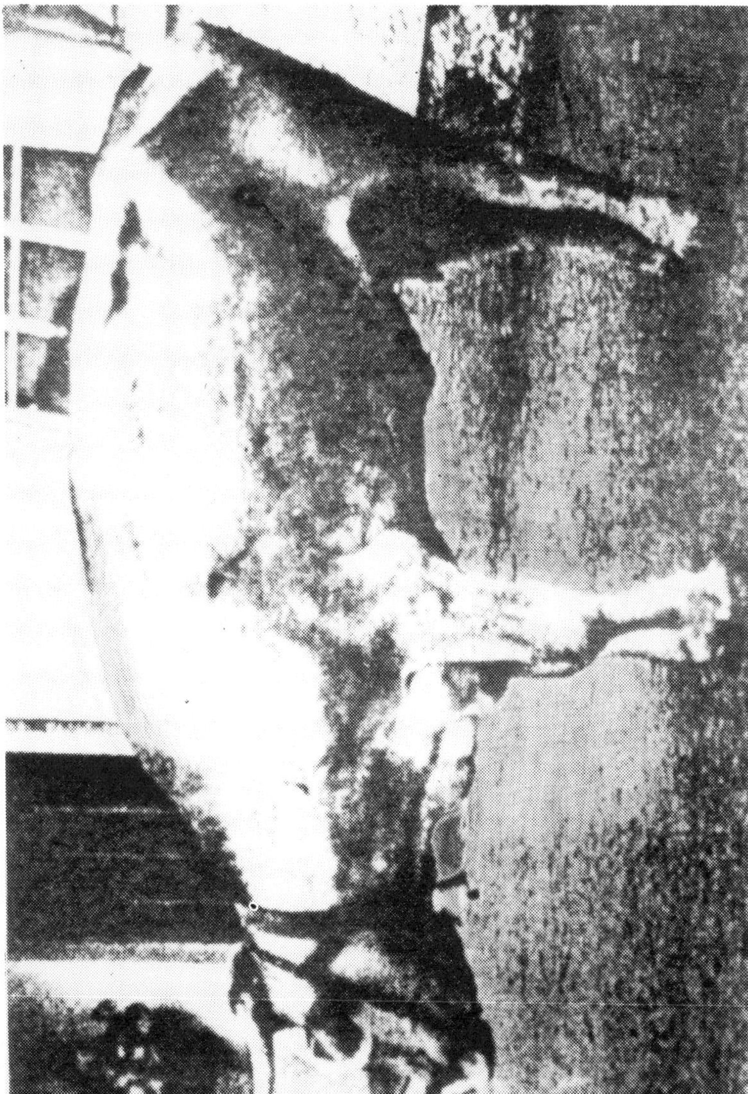

A wasted alpine cow with the curved spine and bent front legs of pronounced calcinosis, caused by feeding upon the nightshade, *Solanum malacoxylon*. Courtesy of the Veterinary Medical Journal (Bayer) obtained through Dr. Martin Morris, City of London Polytechnic, England.

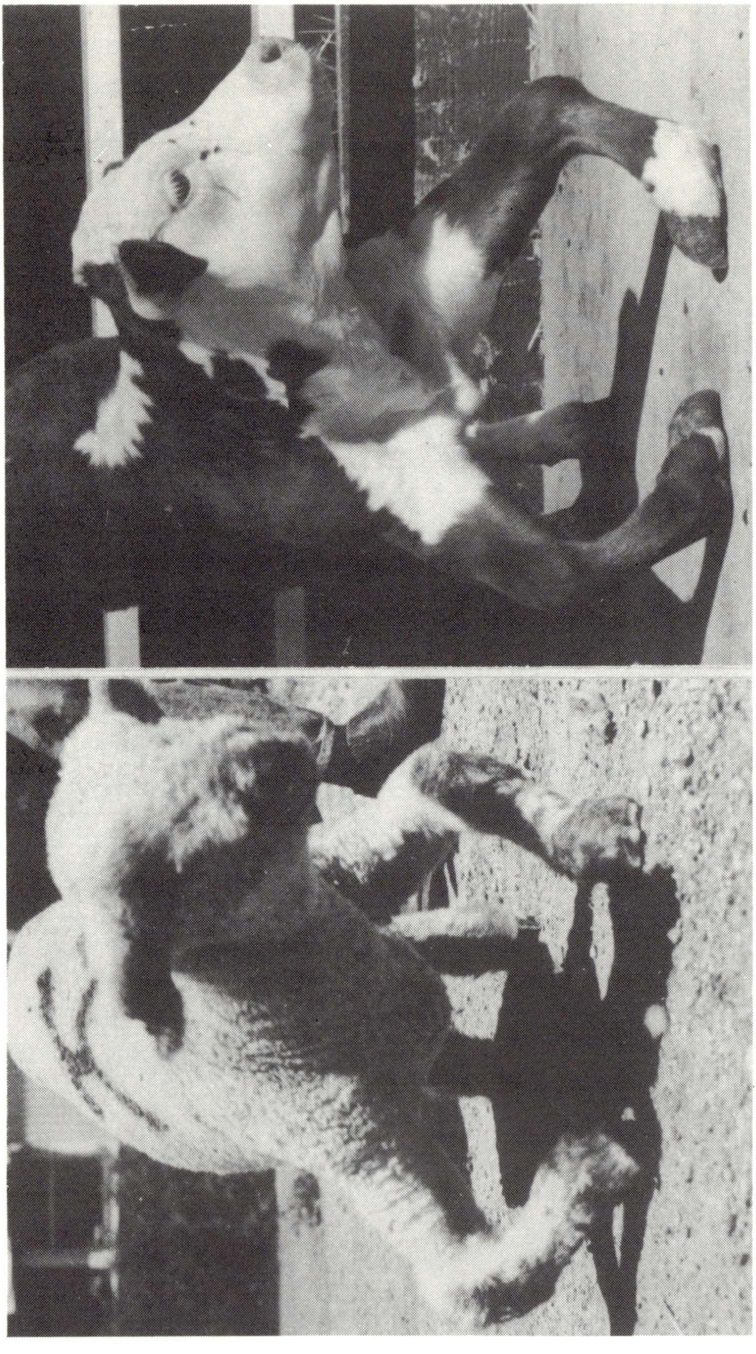

(Left) Congenital deformed lamb induced by maternal feeding on locoweed *(Astragalus* spp.) (Right) Congenital deformed calf induced by maternal feeding on tailcup lupine *(Lupinus caudatus)*. (Courtesy Wayne Binns and R. F. Keeler, Poisonous Plant Laboratory, U.S. Dept. of Agriculture, Logan, Utah).

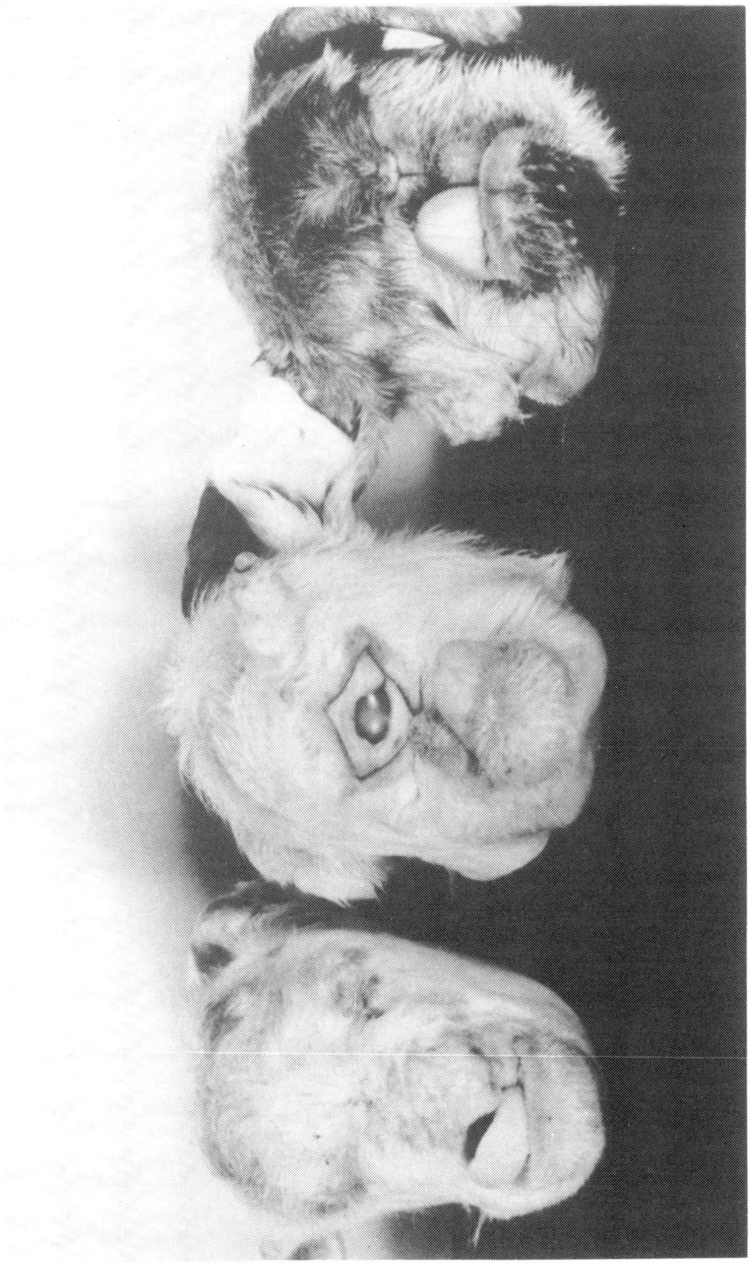

The above photograph shows congenital deformities in lambs ("monkey face") induced by maternal feeding on Western false hellbore of the lilly family *(Veratrum californicum)* the 14th day of gestation. (Courtesy Wayne Binns and R. F. Keeler, Poisonous Plant Laboratory, Logan, Utah.)

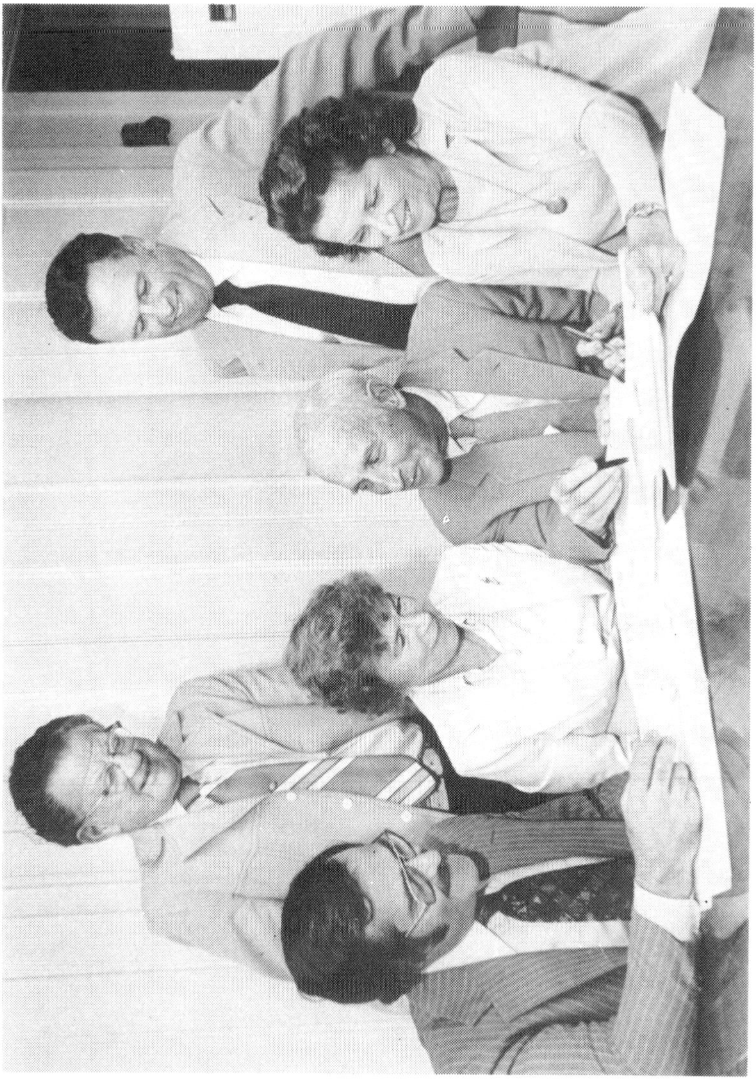

The Board of Trustees of the NIGHTSHADES RESEARCH FOUNDATION are in the early stages of planning here with Dr. Norman F. Childers (upper left) acting as an Advisor. Left to right: Edwin J. Wendlocher Sr., Alma P. Hough, Dr. Ralph T. Reeve, C. Palmer Bateman Jr. (standing) and Emily Osterman. (Photo by Peter Ackerman, The Gazette, Somerville, N.J.)

THE NIGHTSHADES RESEARCH FOUNDATION

Whereas it has been long established that certain plants of the nightshade *(Solanaceae)* family, namely: Spp. of *Solanum, Cestrum, Physalis* and *Datura,* and *Atropa Belladona* (black nightshade), *Nicotiana* (tobacco), and many other genera and species have been harmful to horses and other animals even to the extent of causing death; and

Whereas, other plants of the nightshade family, namely, potato, tomato, eggplant, tobacco and all peppers, except black pepper, generally consumed and used by human beings have been determined by extensive testing to have serious effects on certain individuals consuming and using them, particularly in causing pain and neurological problems, swelling in the joints, stiffness, lameness, back ailments and other characterists commonly associated with and designated as arthritic conditions, and

Whereas, it has been conclusively proved that with the elimination of these crops from the diets of the individuals suffering from the above conditions there is an improvement in health resulting from such elimination and

Whereas, limited research with laboratory animals and livestock has demonstrated that the consumption of the above plant members induces the symptoms described above in addition to others, and

Whereas, it is desired that research be continued on a broader base to establish in greater detail the parameters of the effects on human beings of the consumption and use of members of the nightshades family not only as one of the basic causes of arthritis in its various forms, but also as contributing factor in many other diseases; and

Whereas, the great pain and suffering caused by arthritis in its various forms is one of the greatest worldwide afflictions of our time, and

Whereas, it is believed that further knowledge derived from additional study and research in the effects of consumption of nightshades in their present forms may make possible a great improvement in health in a broad segment of the population.

It is hereby proposed to form a research foundation to (1) segregate the toxic elements in plants of the nightshade family, (2) study on a broad base the effect of the consumption of members of the nightshade family on the human body, (3) the improvement in health in human beings due to the elimination from their diet of the produce from those plants, (4) the possible modification in the products through processing from their present natural state by determination, segregation and elimination of the toxic element, (5) produce new strains of the present products that do not contain the toxic elements, and (6) make the information obtained through the above research available to the general public through printed literature, books, radio and television programs for the improvement of the health of all those who may be suffering from arthritis and other diseases which may be found to originate in the nightshade family.

The name of this foundation shall be NIGHTSHADES RESEARCH FOUNDATION. Contributions can be made, large or small, through Box 699, Somerville, N.J. 08876.

INTERESTING BOOKS FOR YOUR LIBRARY

1. Lewis, W. H. PhD. Medical Botany — Plants Affecting Man's Health. John Wiley and Sons, New York. 515 pp. 1977.
2. Dickey, L. D., MD. Editor. Clinical Ecology. Chas. H. Thomas, Springfield, Illinois. 807 pp. 1976.
3. Rosenbaum, Myron G., MD. Understanding Arthritis, W. H. Green Inc., St. Louis, Mo. 63105. 102 pp. 1975.
4. Goodhart, R. S., MD, and M. E. Shils, MD. Modern Nutrition in Health and Disease. Lea and Febiger, Philadelphia, Pa. 6th Ed. 1153 pp. 1978.
5. Berkow, Robert, MD. Editor. The Merck Manual. 13th Ed. 2165 pp. 1977. Merck & Co., Inc., Rahway, N.J.
6. Williams, Roger J. PhD. Nutrition Against Disease. Bantam Books. Pitman Publishing Co., New York, N. Y. 369 pp. 1973.
7. Schroeder, H. A., MD. Trace Elements and Man. The Devin Adair Co., Old Greenwich, Ct. 06870 171 pp. 1973.
8. Fredericks, Carleton, PhD. Psyco-Nutrition. Gosset & Dunlap Publ. New York, N. Y. 224 pp. 1976.
9. Maynard, L. A. PhD. and J. K. Loosli, PhD. Animal Nutrition. McGraw Hill Book Co., New York, N. Y. 613 pp. 1969.
10. Pfeiffer, Carl C. PhD., MD. Mental and Elemental Nutrients. Keats Publ. Inc., 38 Grove St., New Caanan, Ct. 06840. 519 pp. 1975.
11. Encyclopedia Brittanica. 10 and 19 Vols. (Considerable Medical Information) Encyclopedia Brittanica, Inc., New York. 1973.
12. Church, D. C. PhD. Livestock Feeds and Feeding. Schultz-Wack-Weir 124 NW 9th Ave., Portland, Oregon 97209 349 pp. 1977.

Note: Dr. Carleton Fredericks and Dr. Roger J. Williams have other interesting books on nutrition of people. Write respective publishing companies or the authors.

Index

PLEASE COMPLETE THE FORM BELOW AND RETURN SOON

We shall tell you about what to expect.

NAME ______________________ PHONE: A/C:___- __________

ADDRESS ______________________ ZIP __________

TYPE PROBLEMS: Please check and put a double check for areas most affected: Aches, pains in feet ( ), ankles ( ), knees ( ), hands ( ), hips ( ), elbows ( ), shoulders ( ), chest ( ), neck ( ), back ( ), other ______ ( ), Stomach cramps _____? About how long have you had the problems ______ yrs? Age ____? Weight ______? Height _________? All pills, including vitamins, supplements, pain killers, etc. ___________

____

How often did you eat the following per week: Potatoes ______? Tomatoes _______? Peppers _______? Eggplant _______ Ketchup _______? Paprika, hot pepper, etc. _______? Pizza _______? Do you have a diverticulitis problem ______? Other alimentary canal problems ____________

______________________Skin rashes ______________

Heart problem _____? Kind ______________________

Cancer _____? Kind ______________________

Benign tumors, moles, warts, etc. ______________________

What do you smoke? ______________________

What have your treatments been for aches, pains, etc.? Effectiveness? Other comments. Con't on back of page.

Return to: Dr. Norman F. Childers, Horticulturist,
P.O. Box 699, Somerville, New Jersey 08876.

NOTE: Please report to us every 3-6 mos. by letter to help in our survey analysis. Thank you.

CUT HERE